John Brick, PhD
Carlton Erickson, PhD

Drugs, the Brain, and Behavior
The Pharmacology of Abuse and Dependence

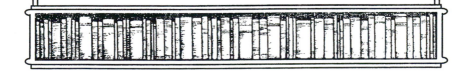

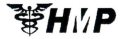

The Haworth Medical Press
An Imprint of The Haworth Press, Inc.

Drugs, the Brain, and Behavior
The Pharmacology of Abuse and Dependence

Drugs, the Brain, and Behavior
The Pharmacology of Abuse and Dependence

John Brick, PhD
Carlton Erickson, PhD

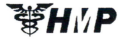

The Haworth Medical Press
An Imprint of The Haworth Press, Inc.
New York • London

Published by

The Haworth Medical Press, Inc., an imprint of The Haworth Press, Inc., 10 Alice Street, Binghamton, NY 13904-1580

Medicine is an ever-changing science. As new research and clinical experience broaden our knowledge, changes in treatment and drug therapy are required. While many suggestions for drug usages are made herein, the book is intended for educational purposes only, and the author, editor, and publisher do not accept liability in the event of negative consequences incurred as a result of information presented in this book. We do not claim that this information is necessarily accurate by the rigid, scientific standard applied for medical proof, and therefore make no warranty, expressed or implied, with respect to the material herein contained. Therefore the patient is urged to check the product information sheet included in the package of each drug he or she plans to administer to be certain the protocol followed is not in conflict with the manufacturer's inserts. When a discrepancy arises between these inserts and information in this book, the physician is encouraged to use his or her best professional judgement.

Cover design by Marylouise E. Doyle.

Library of Congress Cataloging-in-Publication Data

Brick, John, 1950-
  Drugs, the brain, and behavior : the pharmacology of abuse and dependence / John Brick, Carlton K. Erickson.
    p.   cm.
  Includes bibliographical references and index.
  ISBN 0-7890-0274-4 (alk. paper).
    1. Drugs of abuse—Physiological effect. 2. Neuropharmacology. 3. Neurophysiology.
I. Erickson, Carlton K. II. Title.
RM316.875 1998
615'.78—dc21   97-39232
                                                                        CIP

CONTENTS

ABOUT THE AUTHORS

John Brick, PhD, a scientist and educator with over twenty years of experience in alcohol and drug studies, is Executive Director of *Intoxikon International*. As a member of the research faculty of the Rutgers University Center of Alcohol Studies from 1980-1994, he held the positions of Laboratory Director of the Rutgers Alcohol Behavior Research Lab and Chief of Research at the Rutgers Center of Alcohol Studies, Division of Education and Training. Dr. Brick was also the Associate Director of three Rutgers Summer Schools of Alcohol and Drug Studies where he has taught "Drugs and the Brain" and "Neuropharmacology" for the last ten years. He co-organized and chaired the First International Symposium on Alcohol and Stress in 1982, and he is the editor of *Stress and Alcohol Use* (Elsevier Biomedical, 1983) and the author of *Drugs and the Brain* (Rutgers University, 1987), as well as over seventy-five scientific publications on alcohol and other drugs. Dr. Brick is a member of the Editorial Board of the *Journal of Studies on Alcohol* and a scientific reviewer for leading journals in the field. In 1990 he was one of only six American scientists invited to visit and address the Soviet National Academy of Medicine on the occasion of their Centenary Anniversary—the only American scientist working in the field of alcohol studies to receive this distinct honor. In 1992, he co-organized and chaired the International Conference on Alcohol and Aggression and was made a Fellow of the American Psychological Association for "outstanding and unusual contributions to the science and profession of psychology." In 1993, Dr. Brick, a consultant to the Executive Office of the President, co-authored the President's Commission on Model State Drug Laws. In 1994, he founded *Intoxikon International*, a company that provides multidisciplinary consulting service within the field of alcohol and drug studies to government agencies, corporations, health care professionals, law enforcement, and educational institutions. He became Board Certified in Forensic Medicine by the American College of

Forensic Examiners in 1996, and he is currently a member of the teaching faculty at Rutgers University in the Advanced School of Alcohol and Drug Studies in New Brunswick, New Jersey. He currently lectures throughout the United States to a variety of audiences to raise professional and personal awareness about the bio-behavioral effects of alcohol and other drugs.

Carlton K. Erickson, PhD, is Parke-Davis Centennial Professor of Pharmacology and Head of the Addiction Science Research and Education Center in the College of Pharmacy at the University of Texas at Austin. An accomplished research scientist, he has been studying the effect of alcohol on the brain for over twenty years and has held tenured teaching and research positions at the University of Kansas and the University of Texas since 1969. In 1979, Dr. Erickson co-founded the Texas Research Society on Alcoholism (TRSA). He is a member of the national Research Society on Alcoholism (RSA) and the College on Problems of Drug Dependence and has participated in the Professionals in Residence program at the Betty Ford Center in Rancho Mirage, California. The former Science Editor of the monthly lay-language newsletter, *Sci-Mat*, he is the co-editor of two books, *Addiction Potential of Abused Drugs and Drug Classes* (The Haworth Press, 1990) and *Your Brain on Drugs* (Hazelden, 1996). Dr. Erickson is also the author of "Voices of the Afflicted," a regular commentary in the scientific journal *Alcoholism: Clinical and Experimental Research.*

Foreword

This landmark book makes the leap from a purely behavioral concept of the disease of alcoholism and other drug dependence to the neurobiological realm, where behavioral symptoms of these addictions are generated. I am talking about the circuits that account for these behaviors. The boundaries that divide psychotherapy, neurobiology, and spirituality are erased. Each of these are mixed in an understandable way to show how the whole human being functions. It takes the reader forward from the days when early thinkers about such matters began to believe that the mind is physical, and that all concepts, including spirituality, are rooted in the molecular makeup of the brain. This volume makes this more clear, and at the same time does not discount the power of the spirit. What it says is that our thoughts, our feelings, and acts, all arise from the electrical and chemical goings-on in the brain. The book reads like an adventure as it tours each psychoactive drug through the brain. It describes the behavioral effect of each of these drugs, some helpful, others potentially harmful. Not only will persons unfamiliar with the exquisite workings of the brain find this book fascinating, but neuroscientists will get a new perspective of why Dr. Carlton Erickson and Dr. John Brick view alcoholism and other drug dependencies as a chronic relapsing brain disease. What has been looked upon for so many years as a form of willful bad behavior has now found its final and accurate identification as a treatable medical disease.

James W. West, PhD
Betty Ford Center
Rancho Mirage, CA

Preface

The best investment you can make in life is in your education. The second best investment you can make is in the education of others. That is, in part, the reason this book came to be written.

It was never my intention to be a teacher. Most of my graduate training was in neuroscience and psychology and my career path was very focused in neuropharmacology research. I wanted to understand how the brain worked and how drugs like alcohol changed the functioning of the brain and behavior. Somewhere along the way, I found myself teaching such courses as Drugs and the Brain, Neuropharmacology, and Clinical Psychopharmacology and enjoying it. John L. Fuller, the distinguished scientist who developed the field of behavioral genetics, told me that as a teacher, his goal was to produce students smarter than he was. Dr. Fuller was a man who knew how to invest. I think of him often when my own students ask interesting questions.

Drugs, the Brain, and Behavior developed as a result of requests by students at the Rutgers University Summer Schools of Alcohol and Drug Studies, where I taught for more than a dozen years, and from graduate students at Rutgers University and elsewhere in the United States. This book will provide you with a solid understanding of how the brain works, and the ways in which a variety of drugs affect the brain to produce intoxication and dependence. Some drugs, such as nicotine and hallucinogens, are not included in this edition. I chose to focus on drugs that generated the greatest number of questions from clinicians and other professionals who have been kind enough to take my courses and attend my lectures. Their inquiries into the way drugs affect the brain and behavior were the motivation to write this book. I hope that you enjoy *Drugs, the Brain, and Behavior* and will write to me with other questions that can be addressed in future editions.

John Brick, PhD

John Brick, PhD, is a scientist and an educator. That is why I was flattered when he asked me to co-author this book. Those holding PhDs who write understandable books on science topics are to be revered in our society, since so few of them do it.

This book is for you if you want to know how drugs that affect the brain work. It will answer most of your questions about drugs, the brain, and behavior, and give you a strong foundation so that you can learn more. Neuropharmacology and neuroscience are moving so fast that some research is outdated (but not wrong!) before it is even published. *Drugs, the Brain, and Behavior* will help you to better understand new research and what happens with people who take these drugs.

I too am committed to education. My mother was an elementary school teacher, but my father never went to high school. Everyone else in my immediate family has graduated from college (or will soon). For me, the research I do and the lectures I give provide a base of tremendous satisfaction and self-esteem that I could never find anywhere else. Thus, I wish that everyone could be as educated as possible, particularly about new neuroscience research findings, how drugs are abused, how they produce "addiction," and how new pharmacotherapies can help people with addictive and mental diseases.

The latest neurobiological research is understandable and logical, especially when explained clearly. Thus, anyone can learn how drugs affect the brain. These drugs can be the cause of great misery or great salvation. Properly used, psychoactive drugs save lives. This book provides the basis for understanding how and why.

Carlton K. Erickson, PhD

Acknowledgments

I am happy to acknowledge and thank the following people for their help with *Drugs, the Brain, and Behavior.* Thanks to Lynn Gibson and Patricia Cully for typing earlier versions of this book, and Jacquelyn Kaizar for endless rewrites of the "last" copy and final production. Thanks to Gary Leavitt, MD, who provided the MRI used on the cover, and to Karen Gutwirth who, with few exceptions, is responsible for translating my cryptic sketches into beautiful illustrations. Most of all, my thanks to Laurie Stockton, my editor extraordinaire and best friend, who read countless versions of this book with a fresh perspective each time.

Introduction

HOW TO GET THE MOST FROM
DRUGS, THE BRAIN, AND BEHAVIOR

This book is designed to provide a solid conceptual foundation of how drugs affect the brain and behavior. While it provides the reader with a quick reference for various neuropharmacology questions, you will get the most from *Drugs, the Brain, and Behavior* by reading it like a story, sequentially. We begin with a historical overview of drug use and move quickly into the study of the brain and the emergence of the brain-behavior continuum. *Drugs, the Brain, and Behavior* highlights some of the most exciting neuroscientific discoveries of the last century, which led to our modern understanding of mental illness and everyday addictive and psychotherapeutic drugs.

Chapter 1

What Is a Drug?

We begin Drugs, the Brain, and Behavior *with the realization that traditionally, drugs are therapeutic chemicals designed to have maximal benefit with minimal risk of side effects or toxicity. In this book, we describe psychoactive drugs—those drugs that change cognition, behavior, and emotions by changing the functioning of the brain. Our journey begins with the introduction of a model of drug action to understand how drugs work.*

Thousands of drugs are currently available, with new drugs constantly under development. Alcohol is a psychoactive drug, as are, for example, heroin, caffeine, and Prozac. Each one produces changes in feelings and behavior. Antibiotics are also drugs, but they are not considered psychoactive, even though your behavior may change (i.e., you may feel better after they have fought off some horrible infection). Psychopharmacology is the study of the use, mechanisms, and effects of drugs that act on the brain and subsequently alter behavior. Therefore, the definition of a drug varies with its action. In *Drugs, the Brain, and Behavior*, we will primarily be discussing psychoactive drugs.

Drug use is not new, despite the fact that every generation thinks that its drug problem is somehow unique. On the contrary, drug use is as old as recorded history, although effective psychotherapeutic drug use is a relatively recent development. For example, alcohol in the form of mead was popular in the Paleolithic age (8000 B.C.), the use of opium is reported in Sumerian tablets (4000 B.C.), and marijuana was known in China in 2737 B.C.

In the case of psychotherapeutic drugs (those used to restore mental health), if the last 10,000 years of known drug use were placed on a twenty-four-hour timeline, and it was now the end of the day (2400 hours), the use of these drugs began only about six minutes ago!

GOLDEN AGE OF PHARMACOLOGY

The 1950s, known as the Golden Age of Pharmacology, promised great hope in providing drugs to treat mental illness and restore mental health. Many of these promises have been kept. For example, some forms of schizophrenia, previously untreatable, are often effectively treated with antipsychotic medications that enable the patient to engage in a meaningful psychotherapeutic relationship and to function in society. Antipsychotics have replaced psychosurgery, a dreadful digression in the treatment of the mentally ill, but psychosurgery is still used in epileptics and Parkinson's patients as a treatment of last resort. The advent of antianxiety drugs and antidepressants has enabled many patients to resume normal lives in a complex society. Treatment of mental illness with drugs is not a panacea, and some advances have not been without problems. For example, there are side effects, such as motor function disorders (e.g., tardive dyskinesia) in the case of some antipsychotic medications. The unintended consequences of a drug (i.e., side effects) must always be weighed against the therapeutic effectiveness of the drug. This is called "benefit-to-risk decision making," which is at the heart of physician prescribing.

The use of psychotherapeutic medications in the United States is widespread. About one in six women and one in fourteen men use psychoactive prescription drugs. About 100 million prescriptions for antianxiety drugs are written in the United States each year, for example.

WHY STUDY THE BRAIN-BEHAVIOR RELATIONSHIP?

Ultimately, it is the brain that responds to, processes, and initiates all behavior, normal or pathological. We learned earlier that psychoactive drugs alter behavior. Prior to discussing the nuts and bolts of neurophysiology and neuropharmacology, let's carefully examine the basic elements of behavior that you may be familiar with. As behaving organisms we respond to various events in our environment in many different ways. These events can act as stimuli to trigger certain responses or associations. Consider what you are doing right now, reading. For the moment, think of how the words on this page and the meanings that they represent act as stimuli. In their most basic form, the letters and groups of letters (words) are nothing more than two-dimensional curvilinear visual stimuli that fall on very specialized cells in the back of each eye. These cells are called receptors. The human eye has two basic types of receptors, one type for color vision and another for monochromatic vision. The images on this page activate entire fields of receptors in each eye. Information from these receptors is then transmitted from the back of the eye to the optic nerve, which carries the visual information to various parts of the brain, where it is further processed. In the brain, associations are made with previously stored information and some response is made. Shapes become letters, letters become words, words become sentences and, if everything is working properly, some associative meaning occurs and information is transferred from one medium to another (from shapes to meaning).

Your response to what you read can vary considerably by simply moving your eye to the next word to complete the sentence. Once you understand what the sentence means you may continue reading or perhaps be stimulated to ask questions or formulate a conclusion based upon what you have read. Two people may read the same sentence but derive completely different meanings. Similarly, two people may take the same drug and have different qualitative and quantitative responses.

The brain receives, integrates, and responds to outside sensory information from peripheral organs (eyes, ears, nose, tongue, skin) and their receptors (see Chapter 4). However, the brain is responsible for something even more interesting than responding to external sensory information; it is responsible for cognition. Your brain stores each fact, thought, belief, feeling, and emotion that you have ever experienced. This marvelous feat is performed through changes in the functional activity of cells within the brain. Changes in brain chemistry produced by external environmental stimuli or internal biochemical stimuli are responsible for all behavior, including those biobehavioral changes produced by psychoactive drugs.

How does the brain manage all of this? In part, the answer is in the specialization of the brain and the complexity of its neural connections and communication. In order to appreciate how drug-induced changes in the normal activity of the brain alter behavior, let's first take a look at the basic units of the brain and how they work together.

BBB MODEL OF DRUG ACTION

Let's begin by examining how the brain responds to changes in its environment and introduce an example of how drugs work through the BBB Model of Drug Action. Imagine that you are sitting quietly in a room, relaxing, when suddenly a cherry bomb or similar device explodes behind you. What happens? If you are like most people, you will probably startle, become hypervigilant for other danger, your pupils will be dilated, the hair on your neck will stand erect, and your heart rate and blood pressure will be elevated. Eventually, when the danger passes, the effect wears off and you return to normal.

The BBB model has three components (see Figure 1.1): a stimulus (S), the event that started everything going (in this case, a loud noise); a sensory receptor system (SRS) for detecting the noise—in this case, the auditory system but perhaps also the visual and tactile (touch) systems; and a response (R). The response consists of activation of many different systems. You may have jumped, been frightened, felt your heart race. At the very least, your thinking changed. You most likely asked yourself, "What the heck was that?"

Psychoactive drugs work in exactly the same manner. Using the BBB model, the stimulus is not a loud noise but a drug. The receptor system is not limited to sensory systems that send auditory, tactile, visual, taste, or other information to the brain, but involves receptors located on brain cells. Let's think about this model for a moment. Are there any drugs that produce similar behavioral or physiological effects (e.g., increased heart rate, arousal, fear)? Of course there are. If you were thinking of stimulants like cocaine,

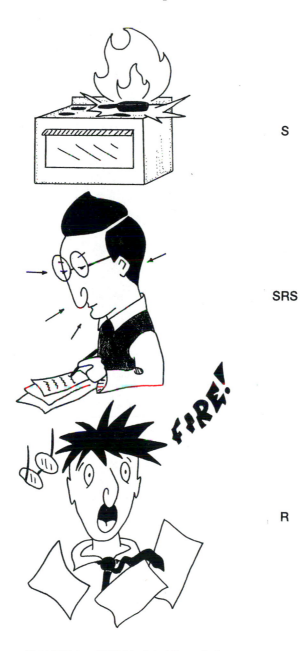

S

SRS

R

FIGURE 1.1. BBB Model of Drug Action.

you would be correct. What if the "stimulus" used in the BBB model was so boring and uninteresting that you fell asleep? Are there any drugs that do that? Naturally there are, and we will be discussing them in future chapters.

The BBB model is not limited to drug use, nor is the brain only affected by drugs. We respond to our environment all the time. Psychoactive drugs change the way we perceive and respond to our environment but by themselves really don't have any effect. That's right, drugs do not make you high! Psychoactive drugs alter brain chemistry and once that happens, behavior changes. Many things alter brain chemistry, not just drugs. People you meet and like give you a very different feeling than people who are "toxic." Both types of people change your brain chemistry, but in very different ways. Similarly, the role of the psychotherapist will never be replaced by a drug. As marvelous as many of the current psycho-therapeutic medications are, there will never be a drug that is as effective or as specific as a good therapist being there for the patient with an empathetic word or gesture. Even so, the skilled clinician produces changes in brain chemistry in generally the same way as the drug. Therapists and drugs are just different stimuli.

Now let's take a closer look at the brain, its parts, and how it works. And for those of you who were wondering, BBB stands for Brick's Big Bang.

Chapter 2

Is There a Brain-Behavior Relationship?

We continue our journey through several centuries of scientific study that progressively lead to the inescapable conclusion that the brain controls everything the body feels, thinks, and does. Consider the fact that by questioning the brain-behavior relationship, the brain is doing something that no other organ can do—it is evaluating its own existence and purpose! People have not always recognized the awesome power of the brain in affecting behavior, or how the brain is affected by the environment. In this chapter we set the stage for this process by tracing some of the historically significant research that ultimately became the field of neuroscience and begins to give us a developing picture of "why people take drugs."

MIND-BODY DICHOTOMY

The relationship between the brain and behavior has fascinated philosophers and scientists for thousands of years. You might say that the brain has captured its own imagination. It was Aristotle who, more than 2,000 years ago, discussed how and where the soul interacted with the body. For Aristotle the question was, How does our conscious mind (what he called the soul) enter the physical body and what happens to the mind/soul when we die? Descartes (1596-1650), a philosopher, viewed the mind and the body as separate. He believed that the body was simply a robot with biological parts that had "reflex" actions. These actions were the result of animal spirits that moved through nerve cells and were responsible for transmitting sensory information to the brain. Behavior was the reversal of these reflexes, initiated by the free will of the soul and mediated through the pineal, a small roundish gland located within the brain. These ideas were simplistic and not very accurate, but they did get people thinking about how the brain worked.

THE MIND IS PHYSICAL

It was not until about 1651 that Thomas Hobbes, a colleague of both Descartes and Galileo, began to describe the mind in physical terms. Hobbes relied upon the teachings of another philosopher, Democritus, who several hundred years earlier suggested that the body and all other matter were composed of small objects he called *atomas* (atoms)—a Greek word meaning uncut or indivisible.

By the late seventeenth and early eighteenth centuries, the empirical method of scientific inquiry was formulated. The empiricists argued that consciousness could be explained in terms of physics and chemistry. Although the empiricists didn't have a clue about how this actually worked, their beliefs were the beginnings of behavioral neuroscience and biological psychology, the scientific studies of the physiological basis of behavior.

One of the many new empiricists was John Locke (1632-1704). Locke believed that experience is a combination of current sensory information and reflection on past sensations. Locke hypothesized that at birth, the mind is like a book full of blank pages. With experience, the pages of the book become filled with information, and associations between information and experience give rise to new ideas. Most importantly, Locke believed these to be physically-based phenomena.

ENTER THE NERVOUS SYSTEM

The empirical school of thought continued into the next century and both received and projected great influence through the work of David Hume (1711-1776), a philosopher and historian. In his book, *A Treatise of Human Nature*, Hume suggested that the mind is not just a collection of experiences stored in the brain, as Locke suggested, but is the result of nervous system activity.

The idea that nervous system activity has something to do with behavior was furthered in the 1830s by Johannes Müller (1801-1858), who wrote a highly influential treatise entitled *The Handbook of Human Physiology.* In his book, Müller proposed a doctrine of "specific nerve energies" which stated that the stimulation of a particular nerve would produce a particular sensation. In other words, specific nerves have specific functions. In future chapters, we will learn how psychoactive drugs affect specific nerve functions to alter behavior.

ELECTRICITY, THE BRAIN, AND BEHAVIOR

The first glimpse of the way the brain communicates information to the rest of the body came from studies involving electrical stimulation. Galvani noted in 1791 that when he touched the dissected nerve of a frog's leg muscle with a rod charged with static electricity, the muscle twitched. Fritsch and Hitzig used a similar technique to show that low-intensity electrical stimulation on the cortex of the brain produced movement on the opposite side of the body in anesthetized dogs. They then systematically plotted the location of each cortical electrode site and the corresponding movement and produced the first crude map of the functional activity of the cortex.

NEURONS AND SYNAPSES DISCOVERED

Toward the end of the last century, it became apparent that the electrical connections between nerve cells in the brain are not direct. Santiago Ramón y Cajal (1852-1934), a Spanish neuroanatomist, developed a staining technique for nervous system tissue, proving conclusively that nerve cells do not physically touch but are separated by a small gap. Cajal suggested that nerve impulses pass from one individual brain cell to the next. This was a stunning discovery that changed the way in which we viewed the connectivity of the nervous system. The significance of his discovery is probably best summarized by Cajal himself, who wrote that he "hunted cells with delicate and elegant forms, the mysterious butterflies of the soul, the beatings of whose wings may some day— who knows?—clarify the secret of mental life."[1]

Cajal's prophetic view of the importance of nerve cells was ful-filled, in part, by Sir Charles Scott Sherrington (1857-1952), a Brit-ish physiologist who was the first to study and describe the anatomy of a reflex arc and who coined the term synapse. Sherrington also described receptors for food, motion, and sensations that enable organisms to monitor their environment and respond to stimuli.

EVIDENCE OF A BRAIN-BEHAVIOR RELATIONSHIP

The relationship between the brain and behavior came into clini-cal focus in the late 1860s when Paul Broca, an eminent French physician, performed an autopsy on an individual who had been unable to speak for thirty years. Broca found that the patient had a lesion (brain damage) in the third convolution of the left frontal lobe. Based upon this observation and others that followed, Broca concluded that speech is localized in this area on the left side of the brain.

Understanding of the connection between the brain and emotion came at about the same time through the misfortune of Phineas Gage, the foreman of a railroad construction team. Part of Phineas's job was to use a long tamping rod to push dynamite down a hole that had been drilled into the rock (see Figure 2.1). Unfortunately, in doing so, he inadvertently sparked an explosion that launched the large iron rod out of the hole and through his forehead. Much to everyone's surprise, Phineas Gage lived, but his personality changed from well-mannered, conscientious, and deliberate to irritable and ill-mannered. When he died, many years later, it was found that Gage's accident had destroyed part of the brain called the limbic system. The limbic system is involved in many aspects of behavior including emotion and is now also believed to be one of the sites of action for psychoactive drugs.

THE EMOTIONAL BRAIN

Walter B. Cannon (1871-1945) was an American physiologist who studied emotion. Up until the early twentieth century, it was

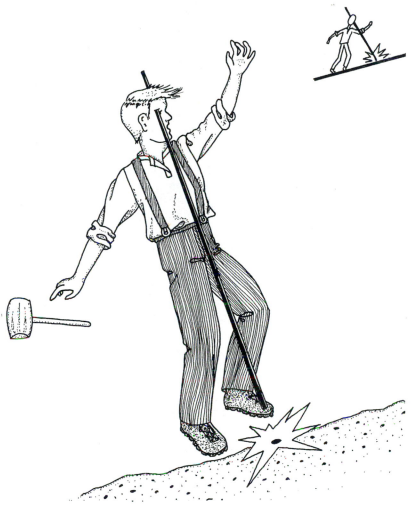

FIGURE 2.1. Phineas Gage.

believed that visceral (i.e., organ, glandular) responses created emotions—my heart is beating rapidly, therefore, I must be afraid. Cannon proposed and demonstrated that emotions are not related to visceral responses such as increased heart rate, as contemporary theorists imagined. For Cannon, it was because the brain signaled danger that one became afraid and the heart rate increased. How did this occur? Cannon proposed that one part of the brain, the cortex, normally inhibits another brain structure, the thalamus, from generating certain emotions, such as rage. When the normal functioning of the cortex changes, it no longer inhibits other brain areas from expressing emotions. Although subsequent scientists have expanded the anatomical parts and interpretation of Cannon's model, his concept of cortical disinhibition has a useful role in explaining some psychoactive drug effects. Cannon also coined the term homeostasis to describe the stability of an organism's internal environment. Changes in homeostasis are a key part of our present understanding regarding the development of tolerance to the intoxicating effects of drugs, although Cannon himself apparently did not consider this possibility.

DOES THE BRAIN STORE MEMORIES?

One of the most interesting findings in the first half of the twentieth century came from the work of Wilder Penfield, an American neurosurgeon. In the course of his clinical work, Penfield found that stimulating certain brain areas produces "psychic" experiences. Electrical stimulation of regions along the cortex controlled bodily movements (motor outputs) in front of the Fissure of Rolando or central sulcus (see Figure 4.3) and controlled sensations from the skin (sensory inputs) behind it. He also found that damage to the hippocampus, one of the limbic system structures deep within the brain, prevents the storage of new memory traces. Damage to the hippocampus also impairs short-term memory beyond the immediate attention span, although memories formed prior to hippocampal damage are not impaired. Although Penfield worked primarily with a clinical population (e.g., epileptics), his work consolidates the relationship between cognition and subtle electrical activity.

WHY DO PEOPLE TAKE DRUGS?

The Neural Basis of Drug Use and Addiction

Over the last twenty years, neuroscience has contributed greatly to our understanding of the specific neuropharmacology of psychoactive drugs. In the last ten years, scientists have become increasingly interested in the question of why people use psychoactive drugs in the first place and what changes occur in the brain to produce behaviors such as craving and dependence. The answer to this important question actually began many years ago.

James Olds and his graduate student Peter Milner were interested in the effect of brain electrical stimulation on learning and arousal. Since some researchers had demonstrated that stimulation of certain brain areas is aversive, Olds wanted to make sure that the region he was stimulating did not produce aversive effects. Using small stimulating electrodes similar to those used by Penfield, Olds missed his intended target and stimulated another brain area, probably the hypothalamus. When an animal entered a corner and electrical stimulation was applied, the animal quickly learned to stay in that corner (see Figure 2.2). What did this mean?

Olds reasoned that the electrical stimulation produced some kind of a reward because additional studies revealed that animals would

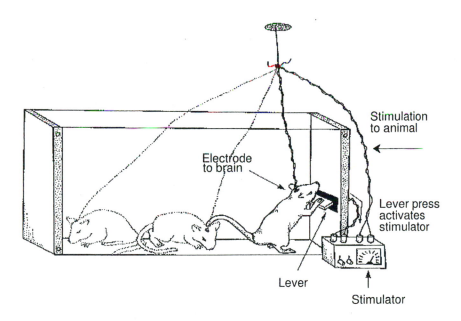

FIGURE 2.2. Intracranial self-stimulation of reward pathways in the brain.

work for electrical stimulation of areas along the medial forebrain bundle (MFB), a pathway of brain cells that connects various brain areas, including the hypothalamus. In some studies, animals would press a lever hundreds, even thousands of times an hour to receive electrical stimulation of the brain. Some animals would lever press to the exclusion of other activities including eating, drinking water, having sex, and playing with littermates. (If you think this sounds like an addiction, you are correct.) Since then, various models of addiction based on neural substrates of reward have evolved.

Current theories about the reinforcing effects of addictive drugs suggest that the medial forebrain bundle is a key site in the neurobiology of addiction (see Chapter 13). It is believed that neurochemicals located in the brain cells comprising the MFB are released by drugs. It is the release of a naturally present neurochemical that promotes reward and craving for drugs. The MFB is part of the mesolimbic system, illustrated in Figure 2.3. The MFB itself is seen in Figure 4.6.

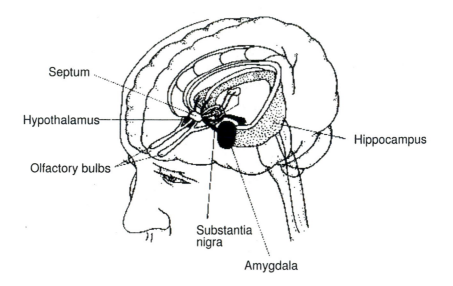

FIGURE 2.3. Mesolimbic system.

Chapter 3

Pharmacokinetics:
How Do Drugs Get There?

We are now ready to begin the first part of our journey—to trace the path of a drug that affects our brains from the route of administration, to the site of absorption, to how much drug is absorbed (bioavailability), to the site of action, and then out of the body. The science of pharmacology has combined forces with the discipline of pharmacokinetics to help us understand these processes. This information helps us understand those factors that most affect the onset, strength, and duration of action for each drug we take. In this chapter, we will learn how drugs get to their ultimate destination—the brain.

For any drug to have an effect, it must first make its way into the body and enter the blood. Pharmacokinetics is the study of the absorption, distribution, metabolism, and excretion or elimination of drugs. Pharmacokinetics is important in the study of drug action because, unless the drug enters the body and makes its way to brain sites and is available to interact with biological systems such as brain cells, the drug will not have any psychoactive effect. Thus, bioavailability, defined as how much of the drug eventually gets into the system and is available to interact with target tissue, is an important concept in neuropharmacology. Similarly, unless there is a mechanism to change and/or remove the drug from the body, it will exert its effect forever!

ENTERING THE CIRCULATION: THE FIRST STEP

There are several means available to move the drug from the outside world into the blood. They are:

- oral (by mouth)
- pulmonary (through the lungs)
- surface absorption (across the mucous membranes)
- injection (into tissues or veins)

Oral Administration

Oral administration is the most common, and certainly one of the easiest, ways in which drugs enter the body. With few exceptions, drugs taken orally enter the circulation through the gastrointestinal system. Regardless of whether the drug is a liquid like alcohol or a solid such as a pill, tablet, or food, the route is the same: the drug is swallowed and enters the stomach. Most psychoactive drugs have no effect in the stomach, but the stomach environment can alter the bioavailability of drugs. For example, Tagamet (cimetidine), a drug used to treat gastric acid reflux (heartburn), inhibits an enzyme called gastric alcohol dehydrogenase (GADH) that breaks down alcohol (see Chapter 6).

Enzymes are proteins that enhance biochemical transformations. In other words, enzymes change one biochemical compound to another. As its name suggests, alcohol dehydrogenase (ADH) is the enzyme that also oxidizes alcohol. Therefore, the bioavailability of alcohol will be reduced if a person takes fructose, a sugar that increases the activity of ADH.

Gastric enzymes may also decrease bioavailability of a drug by destroying the drug in the stomach. Cocaine and heroin, for example, can produce psychoactive effects when consumed orally, but because these drugs are partially digested in the stomach, bioavailability is low. These examples simply point out that some indirect drug effects that may ultimately alter intoxication occur in the stomach.

For the drug taken orally to exert its effect, it must first get out of the stomach and into the circulation. This process begins as the drug passes from the stomach into the upper portion of the small intestine or ileum. If the drug is water soluble (easily dissolved in water) and cell permeable (passes through the lipid membrane of cells), it will be able to move through the walls of the small intestines and into the capillaries (small blood vessels) that surround the intestines. The drug is now in the circulation. Lipid and water solubility are not an issue for psychotherapeutic drugs which have been designed to enter the circulation easily. There are some differences in bioavailability among street drugs.

Once in the gastric capillaries of the circulatory system, the drug travels through the hepatic portal vein to the liver. From the liver, the circulatory system returns the blood to the heart, where it is then pumped to the lungs, back to the heart, and onward to the rest of the body, including the brain. The entire blood supply makes its way around the body about once a minute and eventually the drug is distributed to every organ and cell in the body (see Figures 3.1 and 3.2).

Drugs taken into the body through the oral route can be affected by the presence or absence of food. For most psychoactive drugs taken orally, food slows down absorption and thus bioavailability. Alcohol also does this by slowing movement of food (and consequently alcohol) from the stomach to the upper intestine.

Advantages

Oral drug administration is convenient, doesn't require any specialized equipment or training, and provides a relatively rapid onset for solid drugs—about fifteen to thirty minutes. Less time is usually required if the drug is in liquid form. Also, if the drug is very toxic, purging the remaining drug from the stomach ("pumping the stomach") will minimize the amount of drug entering the system and its degree of toxicity.

Disadvantages

Despite its advantages and popular use, for both therapeutic and nontherapeutic drugs, oral administration is variable and too slow in most emergency situations. It may pose administration problems in older or younger patients. Some patients may not be able to swallow a large tablet or capsule. If the patient is unconscious, oral administration is not an option.

Pulmonary Administration

Drugs that are inhaled directly into the lungs, by definition, enter the circulation through the pulmonary system. When tobacco, mari-

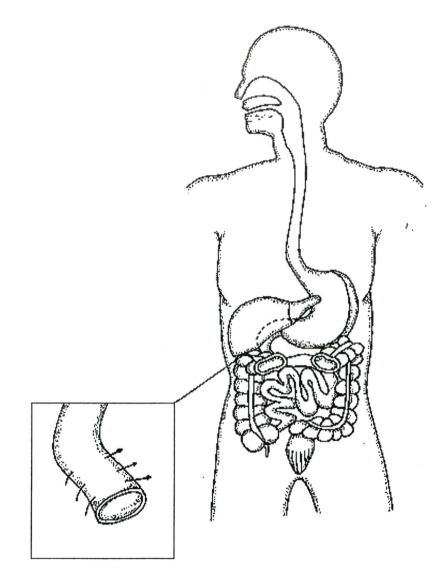

FIGURE 3.1. Gastrointestinal system. Most psychoactive drugs that are administered orally and that are water soluble and membrane permeable enter the circulation through the upper intestine.

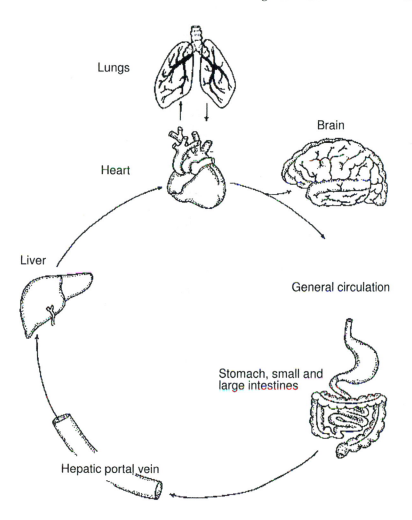

FIGURE 3.2. Once in circulation, psychoactive drugs have access to every organ.

juana, or crack cocaine are smoked, for example, particles of the psychoactive drugs in these compounds (nicotine, THC, and cocaine, respectively) become airborne. Other drugs, such as anesthetic gases (e.g., nitrous oxide, halothane) and inhalants (e.g., glue, gasoline, correction fluid, solvents) are volatile compounds that mix freely with air and do not require combustion to become airborne.

These compounds enter into the lungs and pass through the alveoli (small air sacs that allow the exchange of gases). Volatile or airborne particles pass through the thin membranes of the alveoli and directly into the circulation via the pulmonary artery. Similarly, gases and other volatile compounds already in the blood, such as CO_2 and alcohol, move out of the circulation (through the pulmonary vein) and into the lungs where they are removed (see Figure 3.3).

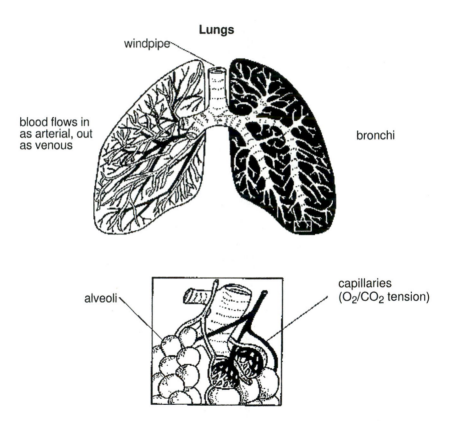

FIGURE 3.3. The pulmonary system. Capillaries surround the alveoli and exchange oxygen (O_2) for carbon dioxide (CO_2) as gas tensions change. As the lungs expand and fill the alveoli, high levels of CO_2 in the arterial blood pass through the thin membranes of the alveoli. At the same time, O_2 passes out of the alveoli into the venous circulation of the lung.

Advantages

Pulmonary administration has two distinct advantages: (1) it is very rapid—some drug enters the circulation almost instantly, and (2) once the source of the drug is removed, no additional drug enters the body. The latter advantage is important because dose-related escalation of a toxic reaction can be quickly stopped.

Disadvantages

As with oral administration, the exact dose of the drug that is administered through the lungs is difficult to control, except in a surgical anesthetic environment. Some drug-containing substances, such as marijuana and tobacco, have pernicious side effects including increased risk of pulmonary irritation, emphysema, and lung cancer. Long- and short-term health consequences of solvent and inhalant abuse are only now emerging.

Surface Absorption

Psychoactive drugs can be absorbed into the circulation through various mucosal membranes of the mouth (nicotine), skin (nicotine, some seasickness medication, e.g., Dramamine), nose (cocaine), and rectum (alcohol enema). The absorption of drugs through tissues in the mouth, nose, etc., is sufficiently different that they are considered separately from absorption through the gastrointestinal system.

Once in contact with mucous membrane tissue, soluble drugs can enter nearby capillaries and eventually make their way to the general circulation. It is a common misconception to believe that drugs such as cocaine can be inhaled into the lungs, when in fact cocaine is absorbed via insufflation into the posterior nasal membrane, where it is absorbed into the circulation (see Chapter 7). Nitroglycerin, a cardiac medication, is absorbed through the membranes of the mouth. Other forms of absorption include: through the skin (transdermal) as in the use of Nicoderm, a smoking cessation medication; and through the cornea of the eye (transcorneal) as in the use of Trusopt, a glaucoma medication.

Advantages

Drugs administered by absorption enter the circulation at a relatively even rate. The use of a transdermal patch, for example, can allow small quantities of the drug to be administered over long periods of time, such as a day or more.

Disadvantages

Relatively few drugs can be effectively absorbed through the skin or mucous membranes, and those that do enter the circulation slowly. Also, the dose administered is not always equal to the amount of drug that is eventually absorbed into the circulation.

Injection

Water-soluble drugs can be injected through a syringe directly into the blood, skin, or muscle, or under the skin. The four types of injection are the following:

1. *Intravenous:* the drug is injected directly into a vein. This is the fastest method of administering the total dose of any drug. The onset of effects occurs very rapidly—less than twenty seconds following intravenous (IV) administration. The anesthetic Pentothal ("truth serum") is administered this way.
2. *Intradermal:* the drug is injected into the layers of the skin. Tuberculin skin tests are given this way.
3. *Intramuscular:* the drug is injected into a large muscle such as the gluteus maximus (buttocks), triceps, or thigh. Intramuscular (IM) administration places the drug in close contact with blood vessels supplying the muscle tissue. Haloperidol, an antipsychotic drug, is administered this way.
4. *Subcutaneous:* the drug is injected under the skin and is slowly absorbed into the underlying muscle's blood circulation. Subcutaneous (SC) administration is also known as "skin-popping." Heparin, an anticoagulant drug, is administered this way.

Advantages

For most drugs, injection provides rapid onset with a precise dose, especially with intravenous administration. Some drugs are given intramuscularly to prolong their duration of action (e.g., some forms of insulin).

Disadvantages

Special equipment is needed and injection methods can be potentially dangerous if sterility of syringes and so on are not maintained (e.g., spreading hepatitis, AIDS). If a toxic reaction develops immediately, the drug's action cannot be stopped. Finally, for some people, injections are painful.

GETTING THE DRUG OUT OF THE BLOOD: THE SECOND STEP

What Happens After the Drug Enters the Circulation?

We have now moved the drug from the outside world—from the medicine bottle, glycine envelope, plastic bag, bottle, etc.—into the circulation. Even at this point, psychoactive drugs have no effect on behavior. Regardless of the type or amount of drug, it cannot change behavior unless it makes contact with brain cells. To accomplish this, it must now leave the circulation. Although drugs can exit capillaries almost as easily as they enter them, capillaries near the brain are different because they are surrounded by special cells that form the "blood-brain barrier."

Blood-Brain Barrier

The blood-brain barrier acts to keep certain drugs and other compounds away from the brain by decreasing the permeability (ability of substances to pass through) of capillaries in the region of the brain. It is the reduction in permeability of capillaries that results in this selective brain barrier. This change in permeability occurs because the blood-brain barrier only allows drugs of a specific molecular size or those that are bound to special transport proteins to pass through to the brain. Compounds that are too large or not fat soluble do not pass through the blood-brain barrier, which includes a unique arrangement between capillaries and cells called astrocytes; the capillaries are surrounded by astrocyte cells so that the permeability of the blood vessel is restricted (see Figure 3.4). Although this barrier protects the brain from various infections (so that we do not become delirious every time we get the flu), most psychoactive drugs readily pass through. Obviously, all drugs that produce changes in behavior pass through the blood-brain barrier.

The transport of drugs from the blood into the brain is not automatic and is affected by numerous factors including transport pro-

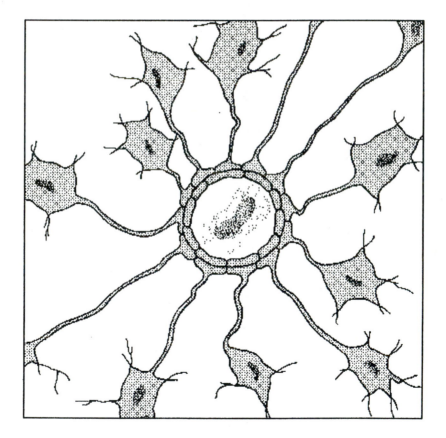

FIGURE 3.4. Cross-sectional view of cells surrounding a capillary in the brain to form the blood-brain barrier. Modified from Brick, 1987.[1]

teins and diet. Diet can be significant since some foods contain amino acids and carbohydrates that may decrease the uptake of certain drugs because they compete for the same proteins to transport them into the brain.

Distribution

When psychoactive drugs enter the circulation, they are distributed through the blood to the fatty and watery portions of the body. Drugs that are lipophilic (fat-seeking, such as marijuana) will tend to accumulate in fatty tissues of the body. Drugs that are hydrophilic (water-seeking, such as alcohol) will concentrate in blood and muscle. Differences in body size, gender, age, and height will affect the amount of total body water (TBW) available for the hydrophilic drug to be distributed (volume of distribution). On average, men are larger and have more muscle mass and therefore more body water per pound than women. Thus, on average, a man will have lower concentrations of drugs in his blood than a woman, even if they are given the same dose and weigh the same. That relationship may change if the woman is a world-class athlete, for example, and the man is a couch potato!

Watson derived algorithms for TBW based upon gender, age, weight, and height.[2] These are the most accurate algorithms to date to determine drug distribution in body fluid and have been particularly well applied by alcohol researchers (see Chapter 6).

Equation 3.1: For men less than 16 years old:

$$-21.993 + (0.406 \times (\text{lb.}/2.2045)) + (0.209 \times (\text{ht}''/2.54))$$

Equation 3.2: For men 17 to 86 years old:

$$2.447 - (0.09516 \times \text{age}) + (0.1074 \times (\text{ht}'' \times 2.54)) + (0.3362 \times (\text{lb.}/2.2045))$$

Equation 3.3: For women less than 16 years old:

$$-10.313 + (0.252 \times (\text{lb.}/2.2045)) + (0.154 \times (\text{ht}'' \times 2.54))$$

Equation 3.4: For women 17 to 84 years old:

$$-2.097 + (0.1069 \times (\text{ht}'' \times 2.54)) + (0.2466 \times (\text{lb.}/2.2045))$$

DESCRIBING THE RELATIONSHIP
BETWEEN DOSE AND EFFECT

The Dose-Response Curve

The effectiveness of a drug in a given population and at various doses can be determined by establishing a dose-response curve. Dose-response curves show the potency, slope, efficacy, and dose required to produce the maximum effect.

Drug potency refers to how much of the drug is necessary to produce a response. For example, in Figure 3.5, Drug B is more potent than Drug C because it only requires one tenth the dose to produce the same effect. This might lead you to believe that Drug B is somewhat better than Drug C because less is required. Actually, just the opposite is probably true. Although Drug B is more potent, it is probably also more toxic. Small errors in dosage of a highly potent drug with harmful effects (e.g., morphine) can be disastrous. For most therapeutic drugs, it's not so critical how much of the drug is required as long as it produces the desired effect safely. This basic pharmacological concept may be lost on "bathtub chemists" working hastily to manufacture illicit psychoactive drugs in clandestine "laboratories."

The slope of the dose-response curve refers to the linear (straight line) portion of the curve, rather than the curvilinear (curving line) section. Drugs with a steep slope on the dose-response curve may have a narrow margin of safety. That is, small differences in the dose will produce large differences in the effect. Drug A (see Fig. 3.5) has a narrow margin of safety compared to Drugs B and C.

Drug efficacy refers to the maximum effect of the drug, regardless of how much drug is administered (or how much drug is present at the cellular site of action). For example, although the caffeine extracted from the coffee bean and the cocaine extracted from the coca plant are both stimulants, you will never get the same intensity of effect from drinking coffee that you will from cocaine, no matter how much coffee you drink. Therefore, cocaine has greater efficacy than caffeine.

Lethal Dose, Effective Dose, and Therapeutic Index

Most psychoactive drugs are toxic in high doses. The lethal dose at which, for example, 50 percent of the population would be

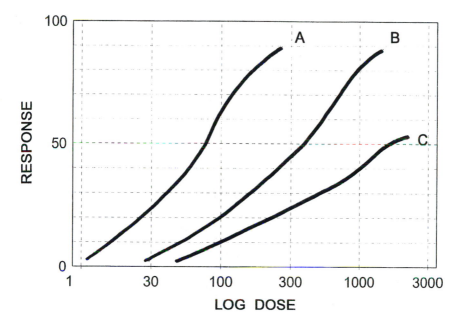

FIGURE 3.5. Dose-response curves for three drugs illustrating relative differences in potency and safety.

expected to die from the dose is called the lethal dose 50 (LD_{50}).
Some psychoactive drugs, such as alcohol, have a relatively low
LD_{50}. Others such as LSD and marijuana have a very high LD_{50}.
Most psychotherapeutic drugs have a very high LD_{50}. Ideally, therapeutic drugs will have a low effective dose (ED). The dose that is
effective in producing a therapeutic response in half the population
is called the ED_{50}.

The ratio of LD_{50} to ED_{50} is referred to as the therapeutic index.
The therapeutic index of a drug tells you about the safety margin
between effectiveness and toxicity. The higher the therapeutic
index, the safer the drug.

Drug Interactions

A drug interaction may occur when two or more drugs are combined. The behavioral outcomes of some drug interactions are often
difficult to predict. Drug interactions can occur through various

mechanisms including alterations in absorption, metabolism, or when drugs share receptor systems. The following pharmacological terms describe the most common drug interactions.

- *Additive effect:* when the combination of two drugs is equal to the sum of the effect of each drug (e.g., 2 + 2 = 4). For example, anecdotally, alcohol and Valium have an additive effect.

- *Synergistic effect:* when the combination of two drugs produces an effect greater than the effect of either drug (e.g., 2 + 2 = 6). For example, both alcohol and carbon tetrachloride, a cleaning fluid, are toxic to the liver. However, their combination produces far greater liver damage than would be predicted from the sum of the effects of either substance.

- *Antagonism:* when one drug blocks the effect of another (e.g., 2 + 2 = 1 or 2 + 2 = 0). This term is often used to describe the specific actions of receptor antagonists or blockers. For example, naloxone is an opioid antagonist. It occupies opioid receptors to block the effects of drugs like heroin.

ELIMINATION

Drugs are eventually eliminated from the body. Small amounts of the unchanged drug can be eliminated through the skin, breath, or urine, but most drugs are changed by enzymes through a process of oxidative metabolism. Enzymes are proteins that are secreted from cells and act as catalysts to produce a chemical change in other substances. Enzymes are present in the blood as well as the liver, lungs, stomach, and other organs. However, most psychoactive drugs are altered by liver enzymes or by enzymes in the blood. Blood flows through the liver, which is a triangular organ lying mostly on the right side of the abdominal cavity. Small amounts of drug are metabolized (broken down) with each pass through the liver.

The metabolism of fat-soluble drugs results in the formation of water-soluble metabolites that can pass through the kidneys and be excreted in the urine. The kidneys, bean-shaped organs about the size of your fist located in the rear abdominal cavity below the ribs, remove waste products through their primary cellular unit, the nephron. The nephron filters the blood, allowing unwanted substances (e.g., water-soluble metabolites) to enter the bladder, where they are then excreted in the urine.

Drug Half-Life

Maintaining a therapeutic drug level, knowing when to readminister the drug, and being able to predict when the action of the drug will stop are important concepts in neuropharmacology. The term "half-life" is used to describe the relationship between the concentration of drug in the blood and time. The time course of most drugs can be described by their elimination or distribution half-life.

The elimination half-life is the amount of time required for the drug concentration to decrease by 50 percent in blood. The distribution half-life is the amount of time required for the initial peak level in tissues to be reduced by 50 percent. The relationship between these half-lives is illustrated in Figure 3.6. It can be seen that the concentration of an intravenously injected drug increases rapidly, reaching a peak almost immediately. The blood concentration first decreases rapidly, then more slowly. The rapid decrease is due to the distribution of the drug throughout the body water and fat. The amount of time required to reduce the initial peak by one-half defines the distribution half-life.

The slower decline in blood concentration represents primarily metabolic elimination. In the example given, distribution half-life is about seven minutes and the elimination half-life is about twenty minutes, since that is the amount of time required for blood concentration to decrease by half (i.e., 50 percent). Generally, most drugs are completely changed or eliminated from the body in about seven half-lives. For example, if a drug has a known half-life of twenty-four hours, it will take approximately a week for the drug to be completely eliminated from the circulation.

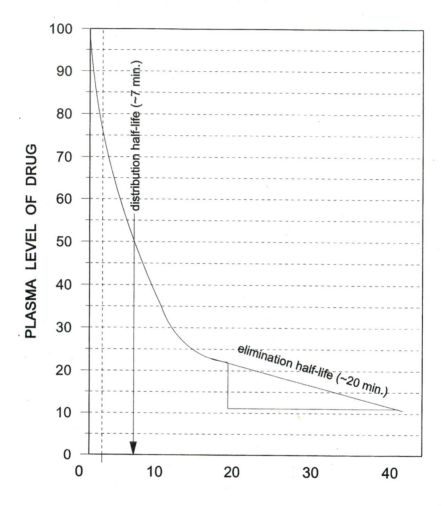

MINUTES AFTER INJECTION

FIGURE 3.6. Distribution and elimination half-lives of a drug following intravenous administration.

Chapter 4

Neuroanatomy:
Where Do Psychoactive Drugs Act?

Since psychoactive drugs affect the brain to produce their action, it is important to understand the functions of various parts of the brain where these drugs act. It is even more exciting to understand that there are separate brain areas for each movement we make, and each thought or feeling we have. Despite these distinctions, the brain is highly interactive with each of its parts, creating an infinite number of movement and feeling possibilities which makes no two people alike in the history of the world.

Neuroanatomy describes the spatial relationships among neural systems, the underlying components of which formulate sensation, cognition (thinking), emotions, and behavior. In this and the next chapter we will set the stage for where and how psychoactive and psychotherapeutic drugs exert their effects.

THE BRAIN IS THE TARGET
OF PSYCHOACTIVE DRUGS

Psychoactive drugs change various cognitive and motor functions by altering the activity of specialized cells within the cortex, cerebellum, midbrain, and other subcortical structures. Learning the basic functional anatomy of the brain is helpful in understanding how and where psychoactive drugs exert their effects on behavior.

The adult human brain weighs about 1600 grams or about three to four pounds. The brain is composed of billions of specialized nerve cells, called neurons. Some of the neurons come together in groups called nuclei. Nuclei have distinct anatomical features and specialized functions. The axons from some cells form long bands or fiber tracts that interconnect nuclei (see Figure 4.1).

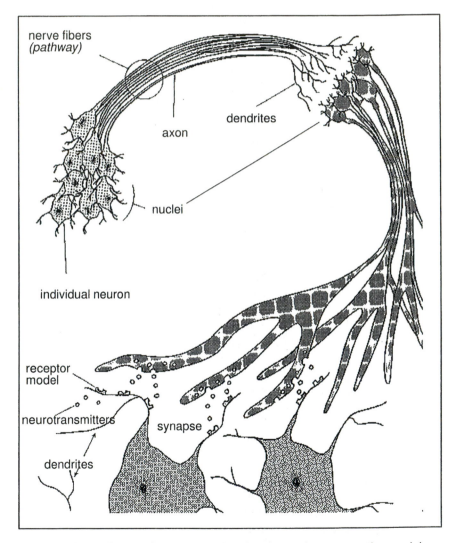

FIGURE 4.1. Brain cells form nuclei and pathways interconnecting nuclei.

Let's get oriented before we begin, since neuroanatomy has its own set of directional terms. Some of these terms will also be helpful in future chapters (see Table 4.1 and Figure 4.2).

TABLE 4.1. Neuroanatomical Terms

- Anterior/Rostral—toward the front of the head
- Posterior—toward the back of the head
- Caudal—toward the feet (or tail, in animals)
- Superior/Dorsal—toward the top of the head or body
- Ventral—away from the back of the head or body (belly-side)
- Medial—toward the middle
- Lateral—toward the side
- Pre—before
- Post—after
- Afferent—going toward the brain
- Efferent—going away from the brain

CEREBRAL CORTEX (CEREBRUM)

Even casual inspection of the brain reveals a wealth of distinct anatomical features. The most imposing structure is the cerebral cortex, a large convoluted structure that forms the front and upper-most portion of the brain. The cortex has left and right halves. These are referred to as "hemispheres." The hemispheres are connected by a band of fibers called the corpus callosum, which passes information between the two hemispheres. Damage to the corpus callosum, which may occur in fetal alcohol syndrome or following certain types of surgery or injury, often results in behavioral and motor abnormalities.

The outer mantle of the cerebral hemispheres is convoluted with deep sulci (grooves) separating gyri (ridges). Dogs, cats, rabbits, humans, and other primates have convoluted cortices, but not all species do. Birds, rats, and reptiles have smooth cortices. The dramatic convolutions of the brain are an efficient means of increasing

Superior
or
Dorsal

Anterior
or
Rostral

Posterior

Anterior *or* Ventral

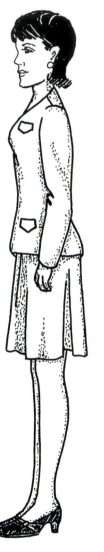

Ventral

Dorsal

Caudal

FIGURE 4.2. Anatomical terms for spatial orientation.

the surface area of the cortex without undue increases in cranial size. This increase in surface area enables a larger number of cells to occupy the same overall space. It has been estimated that if the surface of the cortex were unfolded it would cover approximately 2.5 square meters! The cells that make up the cerebral cortex regulate a number of sensory, motor, and cognitive functions. The functional anatomy of the cortex is depicted in Figure 4.3.

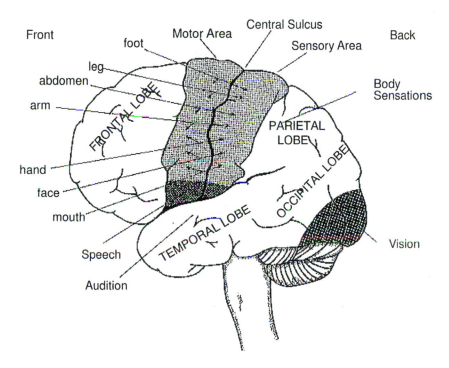

FIGURE 4.3. Functional anatomy of the cortex.

WHAT DOES THE CORTEX DO?

The cells that make up the cerebral cortex form a mosaic of sensory (input) and motor (output) cells that perform a number of sensory, motor, and cognitive functions. Surrounding the primary sensory and motor areas are the association areas. Additional association areas are found in the frontal lobes of the cortex, but here there are few, if any, sensory or motor-related cells. The frontal cortex function is not clearly understood, but it is certain that humans have the largest frontal cortex of any species. Finally, some areas of the cortex are specifically tuned for particular functions (e.g., speech, spatial relationship detection) and are asymmetrically represented (i.e., they occur on one side of the brain but not the other).

SUBCORTICAL STRUCTURES

Below the cortex (subcortical) are numerous structures including the thalamus, hypothalamus, septum, and other groups of cells that form the limbic system. Some of these structures are illustrated in Figures 4.4 and 4.5.

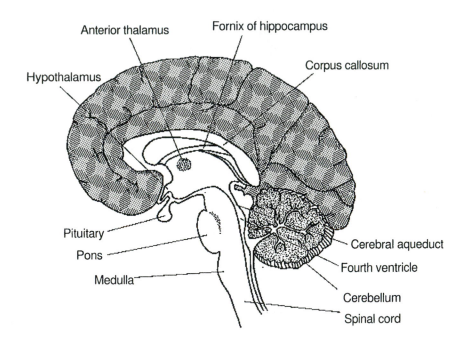

FIGURE 4.4. Sagittal (mid-slice) view of the brain, illustrating subcortical structures.

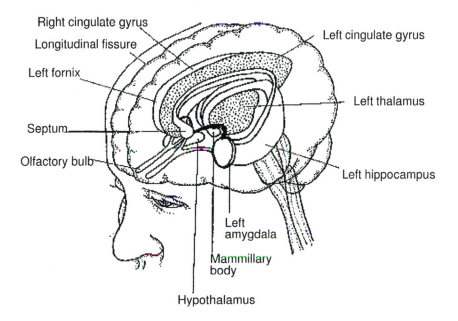

FIGURE 4.5. Functional anatomy of subcortical limbic system structures.

Cerebellum

The cerebellum is another prominent structure of the brain (see Figure 4.4). It has a multilayered appearance and a number of deeper nuclei. The cerebellum is richly innervated (connected by nerves) with sensory cells and acts as an anatomical way station for information sent from the cortex down the spinal cord and from the spinal cord back to the cortex. The cerebellum is responsible for coordinating and smoothing out various motor movements. Lesions or drug-induced alterations in the cerebellum result in ataxia (impaired motor coordination) and other impairments.

Brainstem (Midbrain, Pons, Medulla)

The midbrain is the most dorsal area of the brainstem (see Figure 4.6). The midbrain is positioned above the pons, receives visual information, regulates eye movement, and processes auditory information as well as regulating muscle movement.

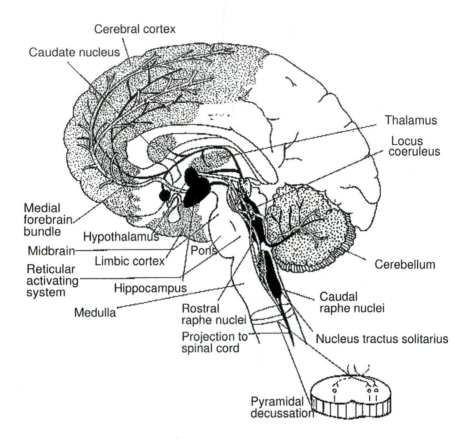

FIGURE 4.6. Pathways and structures of the brain.

The pons contains a number of important nuclei including (1) the reticular formation (also called reticular activating system) which plays an important role in the sleep/waking cycle and motor control, and (2) the locus coeruleus which supplies most of the brain's norepinephrine, a neurochemical transmitter (see Chapter 5). The pons also contains (3) the raphe nuclei, another complex of nuclei that supplies another neurotransmitter, serotonin, involved in sleep, pain, aggression, and other behaviors. In addition, the pons contains a number of crossing fibers of the descending (downward) motor system, most notably the pyramidal decussation (see Figure 4.6).

Medulla

The most caudal division of the brainstem is the medulla (Figure 4.6). Below the medulla is the spinal cord. The transition from spinal cord to medulla is not sharp but is marked by the opening of the central canal into the fourth cerebral ventricle and the absence of spinal nerves. The gray matter of the spinal cord first loses its butterfly appearance and then disappears entirely, giving way to medullary nuclei.

A prominent feature of the medulla is the decussation (crossing over from one hemisphere to the other) of the corticospinal tracts of the motor cortex before their descent through the lateral cortico-spinal tract. It is because of this crossover that damage to one side of the brain may result in sensory-motor impairment on the opposite side of the body. Portions of the medulla also contain specialized cells that control, among other things, the vomit reflex, which is activated when a toxin is detected (e.g., high levels of alcohol).

Thalamus

The thalamus is a central subcortical structure that receives all sensory inputs, except olfactory signals, with projections to the sensory area of the cortex (Figure 4.6). There are seven major anatomical nuclei that make up the thalamus, each with subdivisions. Thus, the thalamus is essentially a relay station where some integrative analysis does occur, but it primarily serves to pass information to higher brain centers. The thalamus also receives projections from the motor cortex and the sensory (e.g., pain) pathways from the spinal cord. The structural appearance of the thalamus suggests its role as a sensory and motor relay station.

Hypothalamus

The hypothalamus is just below the thalamus, hence its name (Figure 4.6). The hypothalamus also receives sensory input of many forms as well as input from all divisions of the brain. Because of its anatomic location, many fiber tracts from lower brain centers travel through the hypothalamus without making connections there. Electrical stimulation or destruction of different hypothalamic nuclei alter (among other functions) weight, fluid intake, temperature regulation, and sexual and aggressive behavior (see Table 4.2).

TABLE 4.2. Biobehavioral Functions of the Hypothalamus

- Hunger
- Thirst
- Satiation
- Temperature Regulation
- Endocrine Regulation
- Sexual Behavior
- Pleasure

Pituitary (Master Gland)

The pituitary (Figure 4.4) is not part of the nervous system, but it receives direct neural inputs as well as vascular (blood vessel) secretions from the hypothalamus. The pituitary releases numerous hormones into the circulation in response to direct nervous system inputs from the hypothalamus. Hormone release may also result from the influence of hormone releasing factors from the hypothalamus. The pituitary responds to circulating levels of hormones in the blood as well.

Limbic System

The limbic system (Figure 4.5) is involved in memory, emotion, and drug effects and consists of a number of interconnected brain structures. The limbic system includes the amygdala, hippocampus, hypothalamus, septum, nucleus accumbens, cingulate gyrus, and parts of the cortex. These structures are anatomically interconnected, but whether they function as a unit or not is a topic of considerable debate. Phineas Gage, whose story was told in Chapter 2, suffered severe damage to the limbic system.

Basal Ganglia

The basal ganglia are important in motor functioning and a key component of the extrapyramidal motor system. The basal ganglia consist of three major nuclei: the caudate nucleus, the putamen, and the globus pallidus. These nuclei are rich in dopamine, serotonin, and acetylcholine and are involved in the initiation of movement.

VENTRICLES

Between the brain tissue and the skull is a protective envelope of cerebrospinal fluid (CSF). The CSF travels through the brain in channels called ventricles. Cerebrospinal fluid is the circulatory fluid of the nervous system, supplying the neurons and glia cells (cells surrounding and supporting neurons) with the necessary nutrients and ions and serving as a sink for the waste products of these cells.

The CSF, however, does not usually come in contact with neurons or bones directly. It is sheathed in tough layers of membranous tissue called meninges. The outermost layer is called the dura mater, the center layer is called the arachnoid membrane, and the innermost layer is called the pia mater. These are the membranes that are first visible when the cranial case (skull) is opened. They protect the nervous tissue from abrupt contact with the skull and confer some shape and substance to the otherwise jelly-like brain.

The CSF is slowly but constantly circulating between the arachnoid membrane and pia mater and through the ventricles that connect the brain and spinal cord. It is produced by the choroid plexus, an extension of the vasculature that protrudes into the lateral and third ventricles. Measurements of drugs, neurotransmitters, or their metabolites are sometimes made in the CSF as an indirect measure of what occurs in the brain.

Chapter 5

Neurophysiology:
How Do Psychoactive Drugs Act?

The discipline of neurophysiology has given us exciting new information about how brain cells (neurons) work, and how they interact to produce a "living computer" so complex that it may never be thoroughly understood. However, we have learned a tremendous amount about how neurons "talk" to one another through chemicals called "neurotransmitters," and how these neurotransmitters act by affecting precise regions on nerve cells called "receptors." As we shall see, most psychoactive drugs act on receptors, but a few of them act on nerve membranes or inside neurons to alter the transmission of impulses. Whatever their mechanism, psychoactive drugs have a profound effect on (usually) large groups of brain cells to produce their pharmacological and behavioral effects.

THE BOTTOM LINE

We are now ready to enter the inner sanctum of neuropharmacology: neurophysiology—the study of brain cell function. Even without the aid of a microscope, the anatomical differences illustrated in Chapter 4 suggest that there are microanatomical differences among brain cells. Let's take a closer look at the underlying cellular architecture and function of the brain.

NEURONS, GLIA, AND NEUROTRANSMISSION

The brain consists of two major types of cells: *neurons* and *glia*. Neurons are a specialized type of cell found only in the nervous systems of the body. Neurons transmit information about other parts of the body as well as the outside world via changes in an electrochemical process. It is the change in this functional activity of neurons that produces all behavior, including intoxication and addiction to drugs.

Clusters of neurons form more specialized groups of brain structures called nuclei, while long axon extensions (see Figure 5.1) of neurons form fiber tracts that interconnect various nuclei. Glial cells are primarily involved in the structural support of neurons and in nutritive functions. They provide the structure of the blood-brain barrier, described in Chapter 3.

Each nucleus is composed of several hundred to several million neurons. To understand how the brain is affected by drugs, we must first understand how the basic unit of the brain, the neuron, is constructed and functions. Figure 5.1 shows the relationship of two typical neurons. You can see that the neurons are almost touching one another, but they are separated by a space. This space is called the synapse. As we shall see, it is across the synapse that neurons communicate chemical information to each other about the internal

2 Neurons and Parts

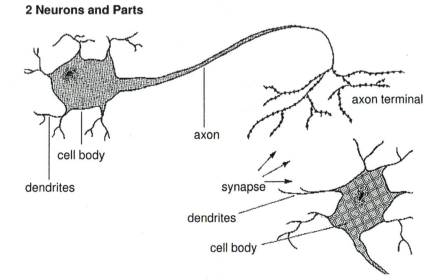

FIGURE 5.1. Spatial relationship between two neurons.

or external environment. In the brain a neuron will make contact with up to several thousand other neuronal inputs, but the human brain has over 100 billion neurons! Thus, our illustration is a very simplified representation of the complex arrangement of cells in the brain.

For a neuron to transmit its chemical message to another neuron, a series of events involving changes in electrical activity inside the cell must take place. To begin with, neurons maintain an electrical charge called a resting membrane potential.

The resting membrane potential of all neurons is negative (-70 millivolts) in comparison to the charge outside the cell. The basis for this negative charge is the distribution of salts and other substances in and out of the neuron. The process of sending a chemical message from one cell to another is called neurotransmission. Neurotransmission starts with a change in the permeability of the cell membrane to various types ("species") of ions.

WHAT ARE IONS?

Ions are usually salts that are dissociated into different charged species. For example, if you add common table salt (sodium chloride or NaCl) to water, the positively charged sodium (Na^+) separates or dissociates from the negatively charged chloride (Cl^-). Two ionic species, Na^+ and Cl^-, each with opposite electrical charges, now exist in the water solution (Figure 5.2). As we shall see, the distribution of ions in and around brain cells is at the center of neurotransmission.

RESTING AND ACTION POTENTIALS EXPLAINED

In the brain, the membranes that make up neurons and specialized biological pumps do a good job of keeping certain ions out of the cell and preventing other ions from escaping from inside the cell. The distribution of variously charged ions and proteins between the inside and the outside of the neuron results in a resting electrical potential across the nerve membrane. In many neurons, for example, the outer membrane covering of the cell keeps positively charged potassium (K^+) and negatively charged Cl^- ions and

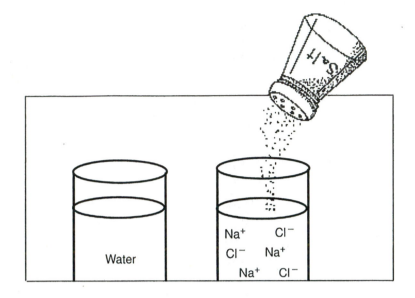

FIGURE 5.2. Dissociation of sodium chloride into two ionic species.

protein molecules inside the cell. Positively charged Na^+ ions and other ionic species are kept out of the cell. This results in a negative charge on the inside of the cell. The negative or positive charge is simply the net sum of the ionic balance at any point in time. Specialized biological membrane "pumps" help maintain this balance of a negative resting potential (Figure 5.3).

Certain physiological events, which we will discuss momentarily, alter the permeability of the membrane that maintains the resting potential. Because oppositely charged particles attract and like charges repel each other, when the permeability of the membrane changes and Na^+ rushes into the neuron, K^+ is repelled out. If enough ions are exchanged, the resting potential inside the cell becomes more and more positively charged, leading to a critical threshold that sets off an impulse, called an action potential. The action potential then travels down the length of the axon to the axon terminal, making the neuron more and more positively charged. When the action potential reaches the axon terminal of the neuron, it causes the release of chemicals stored in vesicles (storage sacs).

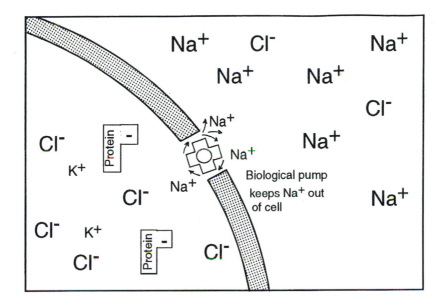

FIGURE 5.3. Distribution of sodium and potassium ions inside and outside a neuron.

This type of neurotransmission is called "ion-gated." The stored chemicals are called neurotransmitters (discussed in detail below).

NON–ION-GATED NEUROTRANSMISSION

Not all neural communication is dependent upon changes in ionic flux. Some neurons have protein-linked signaling in which specific molecules function as a "second messenger" to initiate, amplify, and carry on signal transduction. Some examples of second messengers are cyclic adenosine monophosphate (cAMP), inositol-1,4,5-trisphosphate (IP3) and diacylglycerol (DAG). These and other second messengers may be linked to inhibitory or excitatory second messenger subtypes.

WHAT ARE NEUROTRANSMITTERS?

Neurons and nuclei communicate information about changes in their internal or external environments through the release of a specific biochemical substance called a *neurotransmitter*. Neurotransmitters are manufactured and stored within the neuron and released as a consequence of the action potential. To date, more than forty neurotransmitters have been identified. As we will see later, they can be inhibitory or excitatory in nature. Some of the best-studied neurotransmitters, as well as some of the biobehavioral functions they relate to, are listed in Table 5.1.

TABLE 5.1. Neurotransmitters and Identified Functions

Neurotransmitter	Identified Function
Dopamine	motor systems, pleasure/reward, mental illness, craving
Norepinephrine	arousal, stress, mental illness, learning, sleep
Epinephrine	sympathetic arousal
Serotonin	sleep, dreaming, mental illness, craving, eating
Gamma-aminobutyric acid (GABA)	relaxation/anxiety, alcohol intoxication
Glutamate	alcohol intoxication, other drugs as well
Aspartate	alcohol effects
Substance P	pain responses
Acetylcholine	motor systems, learning
Opioid Peptides	pain responses, learning, eating, "addiction"

WHERE DO NEUROTRANSMITTERS COME FROM?

Neurotransmitters are made inside brain cells from biochemicals that are normally present in the brain. However, the biochemicals needed in the manufacture of neurotransmitters come from outside the brain. Some neurotransmitters are derived from amino acids, the building blocks of proteins. Their synthesis is dependent upon a good dietary supply of basic amino acids. If the diet is deficient, the brain will not be able to manufacture these neurotransmitters. Table 5.2
lists the most common neurotransmitters and foods that are rich in the essential amino acids that form the building blocks for these important chemicals.

TABLE 5.2. Neurotransmitters and Dietary Precursors

Neurotransmitter	Amino Acid Precursor	Amino Acid Rich Foods
Dopamine	Phenylalanine	Haricot (i.e., kidney) Beans, Beets, Soybeans, Almonds, Barley, Eggs, Meat, Oats, Grains
Norepinephrine	Tyrosine	Beets, Peas, Rice, Dairy Products
Serotonin	Tryptophan	Beets, Spinach, Coconuts, Eggs
Gamma-aminobutyric Acid	(Glutamate)	(See Glutamate, below)
Glutamate	Glutamic Acid	White Bread, Flour, Potatoes
Aspartate	Aspartic Acid	Peanuts, Potatoes, Whole Grain, Maize, Eggs
Acetylcholine	Serine	Eggs, Hazelnuts, Dairy Products

Source: Diem, K. and Lentner, C. (1971). Scientific tables. Basle, Switzerland: Ciba-Geisn Ltd., p. 516.

The transport of amino acids into the brain for the manufacture of neurotransmitters is closely regulated. Not all substances can pass through the blood-brain barrier. The transport of amino acids is based upon a delicate balance of different proteins and amino acids in the blood, as well as the presence of carbohydrates. Were it not for the blood-brain barrier, every time you consumed or missed a meal your brain chemistry and resulting behavior would change dramatically! There is some research to suggest that dietary amino acids can provide some protection from stress-induced decreases in brain neurotransmitters like norepinephrine. Dietary supplements to treat neurochemical disorders, such as Parkinson's disease, schizophrenia, and drug addiction, have not been very successful.

WHERE DO NEUROTRANSMITTERS GO?

Once released, neurotransmitters enter into the synapse (small space) between the axon terminal of one neuron and the cell body of another neuron. The neurotransmitter then comes in contact with receptors (binding sites) located in the next neuron. Depending upon the type of receptor that it binds to, the neurotransmitter substance will then increase or decrease the probability of an action potential in that neuron. In some neurons, increases in ion flux that follow excitatory postsynaptic potentials (EPSPs) increase the probability of an action potentiation. Inhibitory postsynaptic potentials (IPSPs) that decrease ion flux in the postsynaptic neuron have the opposite effect—they decrease the probability of an action potential. The process then continues or is temporarily stopped. Eventually, after a fraction of a second, the neurotransmitter drifts back into the synapse.

WHAT ARE RECEPTORS?

Neurotransmitters interact with receptors that are located on "sending neurons" (presynaptic side) as well as "receiving neurons" (postsynaptic side). To date, there are as many as thirty-five subtypes of receptors for neurotransmitters; some are located on the presynaptic neurons whereas others are on postsynaptic neurons. Some receptor subtypes have been identified using specific binding chemicals, whereas other receptor subtypes have been identified using receptor cloning techniques. In the latter case, these cloned receptors are awaiting discovery of compounds that will specifically interact with the receptors. The receptor itself is a special protein capable of recognizing a specific neurotransmitter molecule. When the receptor is occupied by a neurotransmitter, the receptor may initiate a series of biochemical changes that increase or decrease the permeability of the neuron, thereby increasing or decreasing the probability of an action potential. After the neurotransmitter makes contact with the receptor, it drifts off the receptor and back into the synapse.

Once back in the synapse the neurotransmitter may be deactivated by enzymes, contact other receptors, or be taken right back into the neuron from which it came through a process called reuptake. Inside the neuron, the neurotransmitter may be subject to enzymatic actions (i.e., breakdown) or may be repackaged into storage vesicles for future release. As we shall see, many psychoactive drugs alter the functional activity of neurotransmitters by altering metabolizing enzymes or the reuptake process. This series of events, neurotransmission, takes place in the brain many billions of times each second.

It is this magnificent interplay in the functional activity of brain cells that enables us to perceive and respond to our external environment and to ponder a thought, remember a name, or become intoxicated by the scent of a perfume or by a drug.

NEUROTRANSMISSION, DRUGS, AND BEHAVIOR

All psychoactive drugs produce their effects by altering the functional activity of neurotransmitters. For example, a drug may increase functional activity by:

- increasing the release of a neurotransmitter;
- directly activating the neurotransmitter receptors;
- inhibiting the reuptake of the transmitter into the neuron (this keeps it in the synapse where it is free to interact with receptors again);
- inhibiting enzymes in, or near, the neuron that would break down the neurotransmitter.

Psychoactive drugs that increase functional activity of neurons are called *agonists*. Drugs that decrease the functional activity of various neurotransmitters by blocking receptors, decreasing neurotransmission or manufacture, or increasing reuptake or enzymatic breakdown are called *antagonists*.

Some drugs can change the functional activity of the cell directly by altering the cellular membrane or the specialized cell structure around a neuron's receptors. Regardless of the mechanism of action, it is the change in the functional activity of neurons that causes all psychoactive drug effects.

Chapter 6

Alcohol: The Socially Accepted Addictive Beverage

*Alcohol is perhaps the world's oldest known drug. It has histori-
cally been known as a food, a nutrient, a palliative, and (today) a
drug. It is one of the few drugs that does not act at a specific
receptor site of its own in the body. In this chapter, we will learn
that alcohol has almost as many effects outside the brain as
within, yet its use is primarily for its effects on the central nervous system. It is toxic to almost everything, including the liver,
heart, brain, gut, pancreas, and fetus—yet people still drink gal-
lons of it. We know more about this drug than other psychoactive
drugs, yet we still do not know all of the mechanisms through
which it works to produce intoxication and addiction.*

WHAT IS ALCOHOL?

There are many different types of alcohol, but the three most
common ones include ethyl alcohol, (ethanol), methyl alcohol
(methanol), and isopropyl alcohol (isopropanol). Figure 6.1 illustrates the structure of these widely used alcohols.

Ethanol, the most common form, is the type of alcohol used in
alcoholic beverages. Alcohol is a clear, almost odorless chemical that

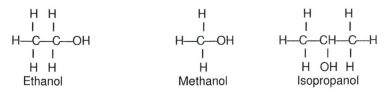

FIGURE 6.1. Structure of common alcohols.

is infinitely soluble in water. It is also a psychoactive drug. Compared to most other psychoactive drugs, alcohol is a simple molecule. Ethyl alcohol is made up of one oxygen, two carbon, and six hydrogen molecules and has the chemical structure and formula $CH_3—CH_2—OH$. As a drug, alcohol produces a dose-dependent biphasic effect on behavior and acts similarly to other central nervous system depressants.

Methyl alcohol or methanol is the type of alcohol that is frequently added to the gas tanks and radiators of vehicles in cold weather to prevent fluid from freezing. Methanol is highly toxic (retinal damage leads to blindness) and small amounts, as little as several ounces, can be lethal. Methanol's toxicity is the result of its metabolism to formic acid, which becomes formaldehyde, a cellular toxin. The enzyme that metabolizes methanol is alcohol dehydrogenase, the same enzyme that oxidizes ethanol in the liver. The antidote for methanol poisoning is ethanol, because ethanol will be oxidized preferentially over methanol. This enables methanol to be excreted with minimal formation of formaldehyde. Unfortunately for some alcoholics entering a detoxification ward (detox) who have consumed methanol, a misdiagnosis of alcohol intoxication rather than methanol poisoning can be fatal. If you work in a detox ward, always determine if there is a history of drinking anything other than beverage alcohol.

Isopropyl alcohol or isopropanol is used in rubbing alcohol. This type of alcohol is used to cleanse the skin or disinfect objects. Isopropyl alcohol is also highly toxic and small amounts, as little as several ounces, can cause permanent damage to the visual system or death. Isopropyl alcohol is sometimes consumed by alcoholics in place of ethanol. The same warnings given for methanol apply to isopropyl alcohol.

WHY DO PEOPLE DRINK?

Alcohol has been used for thousands of years. Currently, more than 80 percent of all high-school aged Americans have tried alcohol and 5 to 10 percent of this group drink to intoxication on a regular basis.[1]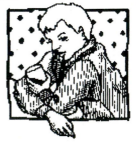

The social use of alcohol now generally includes uses such as a cold beer after a ball game, a glass of wine with meals, or a glass of champagne when toasting newlyweds at a wedding reception. Greater consumption is often labeled drug abuse (or misuse), whenever alcohol consumed causes danger to the drinker or to others affected by the drinker's behavior. Light, moderate, and heavy drinking can be defined by various methods and criteria. For example, the term "moderate drinking" has been defined by the Department of Agriculture as one drink for women and two drinks for men, per day. Thus, moderate drinking in a controlled setting (e.g., not in an automobile) has been found to be beneficial in reducing heart attacks, according to several well-controlled epidemiologic and clinical studies. Prolonged, heavy drinking, however, is detrimental to the heart, liver, gastrointestinal tract, and brain.

There are two general types of problem drinkers, according to the *Diagnostic and Statistical Manual of Mental Disorders* (DSM-IV)[2] criteria: (1) abusers, who intentionally drink too much, too often, and who are making wrong choices about their use of alcohol, and (2) dependent users, who lack control over their use of alcohol in lifestyle situations where abusers would ordinarily stop drinking. Alcohol-dependent people are also called alcoholics, and these people have a medical disease based upon brain chemistry dysfunction (see Chapter 13). Tolerance and physical withdrawal are not restricted to alcohol-dependent users; any drinker can exhibit signs of adaptation to alcohol. The degree and type of tolerance vary as a function of many factors. For example, acute tolerance can develop during the course of a single drinking episode. Chronic heavy drinking may produce exceptional behavioral tolerance.

There are more male than female alcoholics, on the order of three to one. This has not changed over the past ten years, in spite of women becoming more "liberated" and experiencing more stress as they move into the workforce. It does appear, however, that more women are abusing alcohol recently, perhaps due to such social factors. One interesting hypothesis is that women have a "protective" gene, or that their brain chemistry is more resistant to alcohol. Whatever the case, male and female alcoholics can get into trouble with any alcoholic beverage (beer, wine, or spirits) and there does appear to be a strong hereditary component of alcoholism. Studies on families, twins, and adopted children of alcoholics, and nonalcoholics over the past twenty years have shown clearly that about 60 percent of the contributing causes to alcoholism are hereditary. This "tendency to become alcoholic" is inherited and means that 40 percent of the causes of alcoholism are environmental (psychological or social). There are also probably subtypes of alcohol dependence, suggesting several different causes of the diseases known as alcoholism. Exciting new neurobiological, genetic, and psychosocial research is ongoing to further understand the complex causes and issues surrounding problem drinking of all types.

HOW DOES ALCOHOL GET INTO THE BLOOD?

Absorption

In humans, the common route of alcohol administration is by mouth (although alcohol enemas have been reported!). When alcohol is swallowed it enters the stomach. The transit from the stomach into the small intestine is regulated by a ring-shaped muscular valve called the pyloric sphincter. Under laboratory conditions in which the pylorus has been clamped closed or ligated, about half the alcohol in the stomach will eventually be absorbed through the stomach wall and into the blood. However, under more natural drinking conditions, about 10 percent of the orally ingested alcohol is absorbed through the stomach; the rest is absorbed in the upper intestine. In men, a small amount of alcohol is metabolized in the stomach by gastric alcohol dehydrogenase (GADH). This enzymatic activity probably accounts for some of the differences in bioavailability of alcohol between men and women, since women do not have as much GADH.[3]

The concentration of alcohol in the blood is a function of many factors including (1) the amount consumed, (2) the rate at which alcohol enters the circulatory system from the gastrointestinal tract, (3) the diffusion and distribution of alcohol into blood and fluid compartments, (4) the rate at which alcohol is oxidized and eliminated, and (5) the time course of drinking.

As alcohol and other stomach contents are digested, they pass from the stomach into the small intestine. Because alcohol is a weakly charged molecule, it passes easily through lipid membranes and is highly soluble in water. Alcohol moves through the duodenum or upper part of the small intestine into the capillary plexus, a network of tiny blood vessels surrounding the intestines. From there, alcohol enters the hepatic portal vein to the liver and continues to move from the liver to the heart, where it circulates to the brain and other parts of the body (see Figure 3.2).

Alcohol may enter the circulation through several routes including the pulmonary system, the skin, or by injection. Although the efficacy of some of these routes is questionable in humans, they are often used in animal models.

FACTORS AFFECTING ABSORPTION

Beverage Characteristics

The speed at which alcohol can be absorbed, and the amount, may be affected by the concentration and type of alcoholic beverage. For example, some studies have found that in humans the absorption of alcohol is most rapid when administered in a 15 to 30 percent solution and less rapid when the concentration is below 10 percent. Beverages with low concentrations of alcohol, such as beer, are probably absorbed more slowly due to the effect of volume on gastric emptying time, or as Fick's Law would predict, the lower concentration gradient results in slower diffusion per unit area per unit time. In laboratory studies, the entry of high concentrations of alcohol into the circulation may be delayed by gastric peristalsis and pylorospasm. This effect is probably reduced if the person regularly consumes highly concentrated alcohol. Results from older studies indicate that carbonated beverages such as champagne may also be absorbed faster than noncarbonated drinks.

Beverage type may also influence the rate of absorption. For example, beer is absorbed more slowly than whiskey or brandy probably because of the larger fluid volume in a 12-ounce beer versus 1.5 ounces of distilled spirits, even though the total alcohol content is approximately the same. Interestingly, even if these beverages are diluted to the same ethanol concentration, differences in absorption rates between types of alcoholic beverages are still observed, perhaps due to differences in carbohydrates or congeners. However, once the alcohol passes out of the stomach and into the intestine, absorption into the circulation is rapid, complete, and not affected by the concentration of alcohol in either the stomach or the intestines. In other words, the stomach environment is the primary rate-limiting factor in alcohol's absorption, although genetic factors may also play some role.

When the rate of absorption exceeds the rate of elimination, blood alcohol concentration (BAC) rises. Therefore, the rate of alcohol absorption directly affects the maximum BAC. The faster the rate of alcohol absorption, the greater the area under the blood alcohol concentration curve (see Figure 6.2). Similarly, decreasing the rate of absorption decreases the area under the curve and peak concentration, and increases the time from the last drink to maximum concentration. Absorption is affected by many variables, but in the absence of any pathological condition, the two most critical factors are presence or absence of food and volume of beverage.

Food

The absorption of alcohol from the gastrointestinal tract is significantly influenced by the presence of food in the stomach. Alcohol is absorbed much more rapidly on an empty stomach than on a full one. The delay in absorption of ethanol from the gastrointestinal tract into the circulation is similar when food is consumed before, during, or just after alcohol. The presence of food in the stomach not only impairs absorption but reduces gastric emptying time and consequently will result in lower BACs. Although earlier studies indicated that food type may also affect absorption (e.g., proteins and carbohydrates were more effective than fats in delaying ethanol absorption), it is difficult to accurately make pharmacokinetic predictions regarding alcohol levels based upon different food types.

Volume

Gastric emptying is also directly related to the volume of the gastric contents.[4] Stomach emptying is regulated in two ways: (1) the recep-

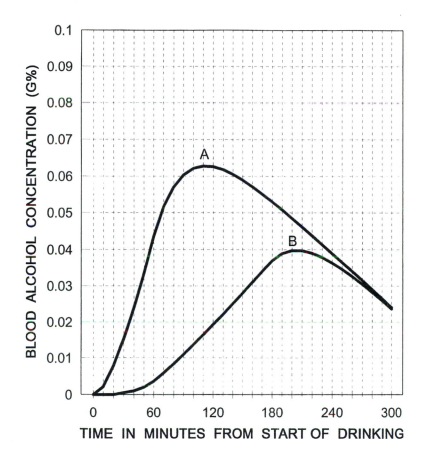

FIGURE 6.2. Different rates of drinking the same quantity of alcohol alter the maximum blood alcohol concentration. Subject A consumed four beers in one hour. Subject B drank the same amount of alcohol over three hours. Both subjects began drinking at the same time, had identical volumes of distribution, and equal rates of elimination.

tive capacity of the intestine (which regulates outflow from the stomach based upon the volume and pressure within the intestine); and (2) volume of contents in the stomach.

The rate of gastric emptying is a balance between the force and frequency of gastric peristalsis (muscular movement in the gastrointestinal system) and the resistance of the pylorus (the muscular valve that regulates stomach emptying). Gastric emptying is directly related to the volume of fluid in the stomach. The distention of the stomach activates afferent vagus nerve impulses from gastric stretch receptors. The activation of these receptors results in a vagal nerve impulse that increases both gastric peristalsis (the alternating contraction and relaxation of muscles) and gastric emptying. Working in concert with the stomach to control gastric emptying, the duodenum decreases gastric peristalsis and limits the volume of matter that enters the intestine to one that can be efficiently processed. In this way, as the volume of fluid in the stomach increases, so does the volume that passes into the intestines and quickly into the circulation.

Large volumes of fluid ingested over a short period of time will result in a rapid increase in BAC. However, the large volumes will take longer to be absorbed from the gastrointestinal system to the blood.

Once drinking stops, the volume of alcohol in the stomach decreases and the slope of the ascending blood alcohol curve decreases until such time as the amount of alcohol being absorbed is equal to the rate of elimination. Then the maximum BAC is obtained. Thus, an exponential calculation, proportional to the amount of alcohol consumed, provides a reasonable scientific estimate of alcohol absorption under a range of drinking conditions. Differences in beverage volume, volume of distribution, alcohol concentration, the presence or absence of food, and rate of elimination, coupled with drinking time and amount of alcohol consumed, determine the ultimate shape of the blood alcohol curve.

Alcohol Absorption After Drinking Stops

Alcohol absorption and peak BAC are important parameters in calculating the blood alcohol curve over time. In some single-dose studies, remarkable variability in time to peak BAC has been reported. This variation is a function of many factors, including drinking density (amount of alcohol per hour). In controlled laboratory studies the between-subject variation for time to maximum BAC following the same dose is quite low (e.g., less than fifteen minutes). Under most drinking scenarios, alcohol absorption exceeds elimination for about thirty to ninety minutes after the last drink.[5]

Distribution

Regardless of the route of administration, once ethanol enters the circulation, it is distributed throughout the water compartments of the body. Tissues with the greatest blood supply and capillaries (small blood vessels) receive alcohol more rapidly than tissues with fewer blood vessels. For example, it may take many hours for alcohol to equilibrate in bone, whereas brain, lung, kidney, and liver tissues equilibrate very rapidly. Since alcohol is infinitely soluble in water, at equilibrium, it is distributed equally throughout the watery portions of the body.

Gender Differences

Gender can affect the bioavailability of alcohol through gastric metabolism (as previously discussed) or through differences in the volume of distribution. On average, men have more muscle mass per pound of body weight than women. Also, on average, women have more body fat per pound of body weight. Since muscle cells have more water than fat cells, men generally have more total body water than women.

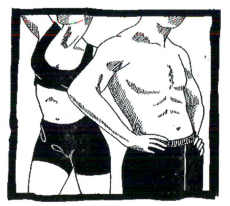

Age and height also influence the total body water. Differences in body water are important in calculating BACs or total alcohol consumed because the greater the total body water, the greater the alcohol dilution.

During the first third of the twentieth century, a Swedish physiologist, E. M. Widmark,[6] studied the interrelationship between the amount of ethanol consumed, body weight, elimination rate, and the BAC. Widmark estimated the total body water, which he called the Rho factor, to be .68 for men and .58 for women. These values are the percentages of total body weight represented by water. Since then, Widmark's equation has been modified to take into account more recent technological advances in the estimation of total body water, placing Rho at about .58 for men and .48 for women.[7] From these assumptions, the total body water (volume of distribution) for a 150-lb. man is given in Equation 6.1:

Equation 6.1: Simplified algorithm for calculating the volume of distribution.

$$150 \div 2.205 \times .58 \cong 39.5 \text{ liters}$$

The most accurate estimates of total body water incorporate age, weight, height, and gender. The sophisticated algorithms to derive total body water based upon all known factors are given in Chapter 3.

NEUROPHARMACOLOGY OF INTOXICATION

Alcohol affects virtually every organ system in the body and alters the activity of most major neurochemicals. This explains, in part, the wide range of biobehavioral effects produced by its ingestion. Of particular interest is alcohol's effect on the GABA system. As we shall see in Chapter 8, benzodiazepines, a class of anxiolytics (anxiety reducers) that has behavioral effects similar to alcohol, also exert their sedative effects through the GABA system.

Alcohol's action is, in part, related to GABA-linked changes in chloride ions. When chloride ion flow into GABA neurons is blocked with an experimental drug (RO-15-4513), many of the behavioral effects of alcohol intoxication are completely reversed in experimental animals. What makes this effect so intriguing is that there is no change in BAC. In other words, the animal is still pharmacologically intoxicated (at high levels) but there is no impairment on behavioral tests that are normally sensitive to alcohol intoxication. RO-15-4513 is not available for human use.

Another subunit of the cell, the n-methyl-d-aspartate (NMDA) receptor, is highly sensitive to low doses of alcohol in the laboratory. This effect of alcohol may help explain the intoxicating, black-out, and fetal effects of alcohol.

OXIDATION AND ELIMINATION

Alcohol is oxidized (changed) in the liver by the enzyme alcohol dehydrogenase, which changes alcohol to its primary metabolite, acetaldehyde. Acetaldehyde is quite toxic and is quickly trans-formed by another enzyme, aldehyde dehydrogenase, to acetyl-coenzyme A, which is eventually broken down to carbon dioxide and water and excreted (see Figure 6.3).

Widmark was the first to accurately describe the rate of alcohol elimination in humans and referred to this using the Greek letter beta (β). Widmark reported β to be about 15 mg/dl/hr (.015 percent/hr). Subsequent studies reported a wide range of elimination rates, prob-ably due to poor experimental design, poor subject screening, and other factors. More recent studies using better analytical techniques have confirmed Widmark's original computation and have suggested that, except in some clinical populations, the rate of elimination is very centrally weighted at approximately .015 percent/hr.[8] For exam-ple, in one study in the postabsorptive (after alcohol) state, BACs decreased at a rate of 14.94 mg/dl/hr (+/− 0.39 s.e.m.). Since the

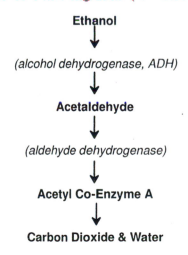

FIGURE 6.3. Oxidative metabolism of ethanol *(italics refer to enzymes).*

range of elimination from this data set was unusually large (6-28 mg/dl/hr), and the variance so small, these results indicate a normal distribution but one with a very central tendency.

Zero and First-Order Kinetics

Widmark's pioneering work has been the basis for numerous subsequent calculations involving blood alcohol curves and making estimates of alcohol consumption. More recent studies have indicated that the rate of elimination does not follow zero-order kinetics, in which the BAC remains constant. At very low BACs, the elimination of alcohol from the blood appears to follow first-order kinetics, in which the rate of elimination changes as a function of concentration. Widmark's β increases rapidly with increasing BAC until the enzyme regulating alcohol oxidation is quickly saturated, thereafter remaining constant. When the concentration of alcohol falls below about .01 to .02 percent, the rate of elimination then decreases and the BAC profile looks like a curved line. Because of the shape of the curve, it is sometimes referred to as a "hockey stick" effect.

Although most alcohol is oxidized by the liver, its elimination begins before absorption from the gastrointestinal tract is complete. In men, some alcohol is oxidized in the stomach by the enzyme GADH. Inhibition of this enzyme by histamine antagonists such as Tagamet can elevate predicted BACs by as much as 10 to 20 percent. More recent studies have questioned whether Tagamet and similar stomach acid blockers significantly affect BACs in such a manner.[9]

Less-Known Routes of Elimination

Approximately 90 percent of all alcohol is eliminated from the body through breakdown by the liver enzyme alcohol dehydrogenase. Small amounts of unchanged alcohol are eliminated from the body through sweat, urine, and expired air. These can be measured in alcohol sweat patch tests, urinalysis, and through breath testing. However, only measurement in breath can be carried out in a meaningful way.

Measurement of Alcohol

Alcohol can be measured in the breath, skin, and various body tissues and fluids including blood, serum, saliva, perspiration, urine, and vitreous humor.

The simplest technique for measuring alcohol is through the breath. This is the method used by most police departments because of the rapidity with which alcohol can be measured and because breath can be captured with minimal training, embarrassment, and no pain. Breath testing is also used by hospitals, clinicians, and alcohol researchers.

Alcohol can also be measured in blood using a variety of techniques. In most hospitals, blood is separated into cells and serum (the watery portion of the blood). When alcohol is measured in serum, the method used by most hospitals, the concentration is higher than blood because of the differences in water content between whole blood and serum. A serum alcohol value can be converted to its whole blood equivalent by multiplying it by about .85, or dividing it by the reciprocal which is 1.18. For example, a serum alcohol concentration of .15 percent is equal, under normal physiological conditions, to a "whole blood" alcohol concentration of about .127 percent. Serum or blood measurement of ethanol tends to be more useful than breath measurement because it is more "direct."

CALCULATING THE BAC

The calculation of BAC is made by dividing the amount of ethanol consumed into the available body water. Body water is primarily a function of weight and gender, as described earlier. Using the total body water (TBW) algorithm (Chapter 3), the BAC in a man or woman can be calculated given certain facts or assumptions, including the amount of alcohol consumed and the elapsed time from the onset of drinking to the time of measurement.

Equation 6.2: Generic algorithm for calculating BAC[10]

$$BAC = (\textstyle\sum_{G\,ETOH} \div V_d) \times [B_W] - (T \times \beta)$$

Where:

BAC = Blood alcohol concentration

$\sum_{G\,ETOH}$ = Total number of grams of alcohol

V_d = Total body water

B_W = Blood Water Coefficient

T = Units of time from start of drinking

β = Rate of elimination in units time

Dividing the total grams of ethanol consumed ($\Sigma_{G\ ETOH}$) by the total body water in kilograms (V_d), multiplying the obtained quotient by the percentage of water in blood coefficient (B_W) and subtracting the total amount of ethanol oxidized at a constant rate (β) from the time of the first drink (T) to a point in time after ethanol absorption is complete will produce reliable estimates of blood alcohol. Similarly, the total amount of alcohol consumed (TAC) can be calculated from the algebraically simplified equation:

Equation 6.3: Algorithm to calculate alcohol consumption[11]

$$TAC = \frac{[(BAC + (T \times \beta)] \times V_d)}{[B_W]}$$

Various slide rule devices[12] and computer software programs[13] have been developed to facilitate such calculations.

WHAT IS BAC?

The BAC is the concentration of alcohol by weight in a volume of blood, almost always 100 milliliters (in the United States). The BAC is usually expressed in grams or milligrams (mg) of pure ethanol per 100 milliliters (ml) of whole blood or serum. The following BAC nomenclatures are identical:

.10% = .10 grams per 100 ml of blood (%) =
100 mg/dl = 100 mg%
where dl = deciliter, or 100 ml

BIOBEHAVIORAL EFFECTS
OF ALCOHOL INTOXICATION

Alcohol is generally classified as a central nervous system depressant. It produces a dose-dependent decrease in cognitive and motor functioning. As BACs rise, the signs and symptoms of impairment increase in number and intensity.

The behavioral symptoms associated with alcohol intoxication may include loss of fine and gross motor control (e.g., hand-eye coordination, ability to stand, walk, and/or balance, reaction time), changes in speech (articulation, richness, coherence, and volubility), and a decrease in cognitive abilities and good judgment.

In most drinkers, as the BAC increases toward 100 mg/dl (.10 percent), it becomes increasingly difficult to perform various complex psychomotor tests, including tasks such as driving. However, it is difficult, in the absence of specific testing, to reliably observe and identify symptoms of alcohol intoxication until BACs reach 150 mg/dl (.15 percent). At that level or more, the majority of people will show signs or symptoms of impairment due to alcohol intoxication, even in the absence of specific testing.

DRIVING AND OTHER COMPLEX TASKS IN WHICH ATTENTION IS DIVIDED

One of the most pronounced effects of alcohol is on divided attention tasks (see Figure 6.4). For example, operating a motor vehicle requires the driver to attend to and remember many tasks. Alcohol intoxication may interfere with the ability to remember to wear a seat belt, turn on driving lights and/or directional signals, attend simultaneously to other vehicles, pedestrians, traffic control devices, road markings, hazards, or signs, and to control lane position, speed, make estimates of time and distance, etc. At high BACs the performance of these skills is further hampered by analgesia and impaired feedback from tactile (touch) receptors in the skin. (This type of feedback is called proprioception.)

Pedestrians are also affected. They must divide their attention among many different tasks. When sober, most of these tasks are performed without difficulty or conscious effort. However, alcohol intoxication may interfere with the ability to walk, in which it is necessary to: lift the foot, flex the foot, step forward, rotate the hip, redistribute the weight to the loadbearing leg, and repeat this sequence, while also allowing for changes in the road surface, elevation, etc. Alcohol intoxication also interferes with the ability to bal-

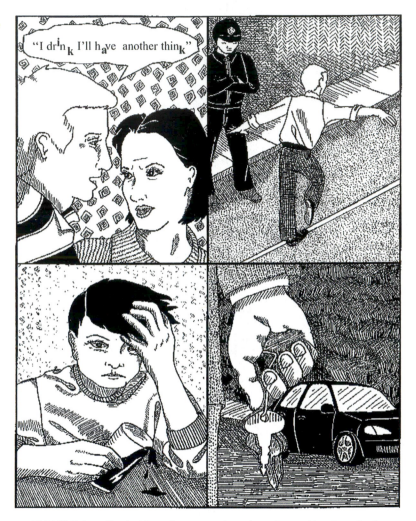

FIGURE 6.4. Alcohol impairs many domains of cognitive functioning.

ance, attend simultaneously to traffic control devices, signs, road markings, road or walkway hazards, or to monitor traffic and other vehicles, make estimations of time, distance and speed, etc.

When an intoxicated individual must simultaneously attend to the many components involved in walking and to highway, roadway, or structural challenges (i.e., has divided attention), that person is at increased risk for an accident. For these reasons, at a BAC of 100 mg/dl, most individuals will be at significant risk for an accident due to the intoxicating effects of alcohol. At BACs of 150 mg/dl and more, a significant risk for a fatal pedestrian accident exists. Alcohol intoxication is also a significant predictor of suicide.

All drinkers acquire some tolerance to the effects of alcohol. A tolerant drinker will require much more alcohol than a nontolerant drinker to obtain the same effect. Chronic heavy drinkers may become exceptionally tolerant to the intoxicating effects of alcohol. An amount of alcohol that would cause observable intoxication in most drinkers may have little or no such effect in a chronic heavy drinker. Such individuals often consume significant amounts of alcohol without showing signs of intoxication.

People rarely look visibly intoxicated at BACs that produce impairment in complex divided attention tasks, such as driving. Most drinkers will not appear visibly intoxicated (impaired) at BACs of .10 percent (the current legal limit in most states), unless they are given specific tests. The reality is that virtually all drinkers are at increased risk for an accident at BACs that do not produce visible intoxication (Figure 6.5). Some states now have instituted a BAC of 0.08 percent as legal evidence of drunk driving, and many foreign countries use .05 percent as the legal limit, even though most fatal accidents occur when the BAC is greater than .15 percent. The scientific evidence (although incomplete) suggests that a lower DWI limit (e.g., less than or equal to .08 percent) may be justified.

ALCOHOL AND THE FETUS

It was not until about 1968 that scientists observed and documented a constellation of birth defects (fetal alcohol syndrome, FAS) in the offspring of women who drank heavily during pregnancy. Children with FAS (see Figure 6.6) have distinct physical features, including craniofacial defects (e.g., small head circumference, epicanthal folds, small palpebral fissures, maxillary hypoplasia, thin upper lip) and overall are smaller in size than non–alcohol exposed infants. About half of all FAS children have some degree of mental retardation (IQs of less than 70). Although physical features of the syndrome become less distinct with age, the psychological

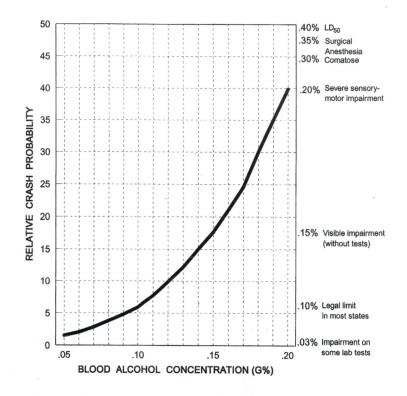

FIGURE 6.5. Relationship between BAC, relative accident risk, and behavior. Some effects may vary due to individual differences. Modified from Brick (1994).[14]

characteristics (e.g., poor interpersonal relationships, poor impulse control, mental retardation) do not diminish.

Conservative estimates indicate that each day about three to four children are born with FAS in the United States. About ten to fifteen times as many children are born with a diagnosis of fetal alcohol effects (FAE), a term used when the full-blown problems of FAS are not present, but alcohol use during pregnancy and behavioral disorders have been confirmed. In experimental animals, large single doses of alcohol can produce many of the features of FAS, but no such cases of binge drinking-caused FAS have been documented in humans. Most

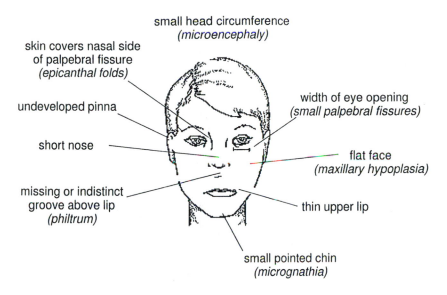

FIGURE 6.6. Craniofacial characteristics of FAS.

medical authorities on the subject agree that there is no known safe dose of alcohol that can be consumed during pregnancy.

OTHER MEDICAL CONSEQUENCES OF ALCOHOL

Chronic heavy drinking can produce liver damage (e.g., fatty liver, cirrhosis), cardiovascular diseases (e.g., heart disease, hypotension), brain damage (cerebellum degeneration, enlarged ventricles), peripheral nerve damage (e.g., neuropathies, paresthesias), neurological damage (cognitive and memory impairment), and motor disorders (gait).

Withdrawal

Untreated alcohol withdrawal can range from flu-like symptoms to a life threatening event. Early stage withdrawal, about one to four days after abstinence, include: transient visual or tactile hallucinations, irritability, tremor, insomnia, tachycardia, and convulsions. Late state (one to seven days after abstinence) withdrawal symptoms include persistent hallucinations, cognitive impairment, agitation, delirium tremens, hypotension, diaphoresis (weating), and fever.

Chapter 7

Cocaine and Other Stimulants: Drugs That Make Us High

Stimulants such as cocaine have been glamorized by many and feared by some. Cocaine, considered by most to be the world's most addicting drug, is a powerful euphoriant that has a legal use as a local anesthetic. Its extreme abuse potential, however, causes it to be a major problem from the upper middle class (where the powder is mainly used), to the crime-ridden economically-disadvantaged population (where it is mainly used as crack or freebase). Amphetamines are legal prescription drugs that have gone awry in over-prescribed uses for attention-deficit hyperactivity disorder (ADHD), obesity, and narcolepsy. Even street users find that amphetamine and its derivatives satisfy their hunger when they cannot obtain other drugs. We now begin our study of the mostly illegal stimulants, cocaine and amphetamines, but end with caffeine, a legal stimulant overused by a multitude of the population even though it is not addicting in the strict sense. As we shall see, each of these drugs stimulates the nervous system in somewhat different ways.

Stimulants are drugs that produce effects similar, and in some cases identical, to the normal actions of the sympathetic nervous system. Because of the ability of these drugs to increase heart rate and blood pressure, dilate the pupils, and increase arousal, they are sometimes referred to as sympathomimetics. These drugs often have a remarkable molecular similarity to neurotransmitters and hormones outside the brain, which explains their ability to mimic peripheral and central nervous system effects. Figure 7.1 shows the

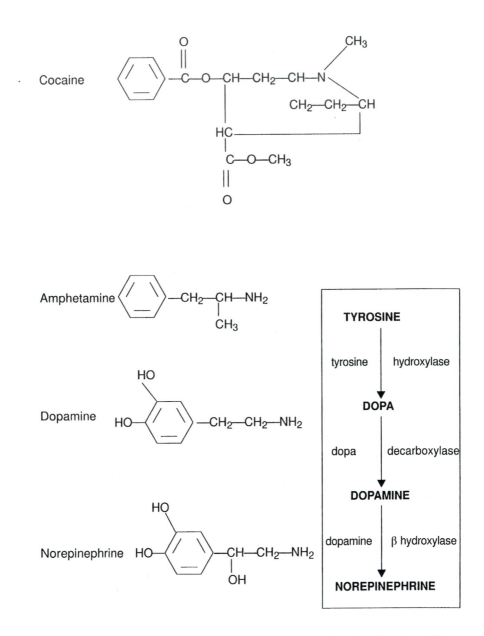

FIGURE 7.1. Biochemical structures of various sympathomimetics. Insert illustrates biosynthesis of catecholamines.

molecular structures of cocaine, amphetamine, and two neurotransmitters.

The three most commonly used stimulants, and those that will be
discussed here, are cocaine, amphetamine, and caffeine, although
other drugs (e.g., nicotine) also have stimulating effects.

COCAINE

Cocaine is a powerful, but short-acting, central nervous system
stimulant. Street cocaine goes by many names, including coke, C,
snow, blow, toot, nose candy, and the lady, but they all refer to one
drug: cocaine hydrochloride.

Cocaine is not a new drug. South American Indians have chewed
coca leaves for their psychoactive effects for thousands of years and
its use is an intricate part of their culture. In Europe at the turn of the
century, it was recommended for travelers, hikers, and soldiers
because it suppresses appetite and is a mild stimulant.

In the United States cocaine was used in soft drinks (Coca-Cola)
and wines for many years, until 1914 when its use was stopped by the
Harrison Narcotic Act. Cocaine's legal therapeutic use today is
restricted to local anesthesia for eye surgery. Today's cocaine is much
more potent and has a greater potential for abuse, addiction, and toxicity. The abuse of cocaine has increased dramatically in the last decade.
Among high school seniors and college-aged students responding to a
large-scale national survey, about 10 to 15 percent have used cocaine at
least once and about one out of twenty young adults use cocaine
monthly. There is evidence that in the last few years, the perception of
cocaine as harmful is increasing among young adults and its use is
decreasing. Crack use, although low (1 percent of young adults report
use in the past month), is increasing.[1]

From Leaf to Grief

Cocaine is extracted from the leaves of *Erythroxylon coca*, a
shrub-like tree that grows abundantly in the mountains of Peru,
Colombia, and Bolivia. Oral administration produces psychoactive
effects. The chewing of coca leaves has a social use similar to "cof-

fee breaks" in this country. Small amounts of cocaine are extracted into the saliva and absorbed into the circulation. Very little is known about coca leaf abuse or addiction in this culture and it is difficult to diagnose and compare cocaine-related problems between industrial-technocratic societies and agrarian societies. In any event, the chewing of coca leaves is not popular in the United States, where the leaf form of the plant is rarely seen. In the United States and in many other countries, the most common form of cocaine is a white powdery crystal, or the harder, chunky, off-white form of cocaine called crack. Crack is so named because of the "crackling" sound it makes when smoked.

There is a significant difference in potency and effect between the leaf and either pharmaceutical or street grade cocaine. That difference begins with an extraction process. The waxy elliptical leaves of the plant are soaked in kerosene and sulfuric acid to form a coca paste (cocaine sulfate). The addition of hydrochloric acid forms powdery flakes or rocks of cocaine hydrochloride. When cocaine is chemically altered by removing its chemical base, crack is formed.

All of the consequences of cocaine use also apply to crack use. This very addictive, smokable, freebase form has many names including base, rock, Roxanne, and gravel. "Pasta" or "bazooka" are forms of freebase that come from an intermediate step in cocaine manufacture. Generally, these forms of cocaine contain toxic solvents such as kerosene or gasoline.

"Baseballing" is a another method used to convert cocaine hydrochloride to freebase cocaine. It produces a very pure form of the drug, but the conversion process is dangerous and involves the use of highly flammable chemicals such as ether. The "dirty basing" method adds fewer toxic chemicals but does not remove the impurities in the cocaine.

Administration

There are three common routes for administering cocaine:

1. *Insufflation:* In this country, the most common route of administration is "insufflation," more commonly known as "snorting." During insufflation, one end of a straw, rolled dollar bill,

etc., is placed in the nose while the other moves along a pre-pared "line" of the drug. The user closes off the opposite nostril and inhales quickly and deeply, drawing the powder up the tube and into the posterior portion of the nasal septum. Within about three minutes, the drug is absorbed through the nasal epithelium, into the circulation, and then to the brain.

2. *Injection:* Cocaine hydrochloride is water soluble and can be mixed with water (or some other fluid) and injected through a needle with a syringe. The most effective and common type of injection is intravenous. When injected intravenously, the drug gets to the brain in about fifteen seconds and the "rush" begins.

3. *Pulmonary:* Crack cocaine is smoked in a pipe. It is absorbed immediately into the blood supply through the lungs. The rush from smoking crack cocaine is very rapid, as the drug gets to the brain in about five seconds. Paste may also be smoked in a cigarette or joint, although this is not very common in the United States.

Half-Life

Cocaine hydrochloride is rapidly metabolized and eliminated. The elimination half-life is approximately one hour. Although the half-lives for different routes of administration may vary, they have not yet been studied.

Pharmacological Action

Cocaine acts to block the reuptake of brain dopamine and (to a lesser extent) serotonin. Earlier studies also demonstrated that cocaine increased the release of dopamine and inhibited the reup-take of norepinephrine, but its primary mechanism of action now appears to be blocking the reuptake of dopamine.[2]

The Cocaine High

Cocaine, perhaps more than any other addicting drug, produces its effects by stimulating mesolimbic dopamine reward/pleasure pathways (see Chapter 13). The "desirable" behavioral effects of cocaine intoxication include euphoria, a sense of omnipotence, hypervigilance, well-being, and endless energy. Although these subjective states are well-defined and, according to many users, unparalleled in the quality of the "high," the effects are very short-lived following a single dose. Peak cocaine (hydrochloride) effects occur in about fifteen to thirty minutes with some lingering effects for up to about an hour. Crack cocaine effects are shorter—five to ten minutes. The subjective effects of the high then diminish quickly, until more drug is administered.

Physically, cocaine relieves fatigue, increases heart rate, respiration, temperature, and blood pressure, causes pupil dilation (mydriasis), and is a local anesthetic.

Some cocaine users drink alcohol to produce various types of cognitive performance changes. With chronic use of both drugs, alcohol seems to increase the body's sensitivity to cocaine. This effect may be due to the production of cocaethylene, which has a half-life almost three times longer than cocaine. Cocaethylene also appears to block the reuptake of dopamine to produce its pharmacological effects and may exacerbate the effects of alcohol.

HARMFUL SIDE EFFECTS OF COCAINE

Psychological Consequences

As the drug wears off, the euphoria is followed by a physiological and psychological depression called a "crash." The crash includes rebound sleep, clinical depression, and autonomic dysfunction. About 95 percent of the symptoms are emotional, not physical. Crack smokers as well as intravenous cocaine "shooters" report that after the rush there is an intense craving for more drug. These effects are probably associated with the depletion of dopamine and serotonin caused by using the drug over a prolonged period of time.

While intoxicated, many people engage in repetitive, almost compulsive motor activity such as rearranging furniture or the contents of pocketbooks, wallets, etc. Some users state that resisting such urges is uncomfortable and aversive.

Heart Attacks, Convulsions, and Death

Cocaine's sympathomimetic effects include increases in heart rate and blood pressure (it constricts blood vessels). One intravenous cocaine addict reported that he knew when he had good cocaine because he felt as though his heart was going to explode through his chest. Some of these biomedical consequences increase the risk of stroke due to hypertension/weakened blood vessels, heart attack from severe tachycardia, and seizures from excessive central nervous system stimulation.

Fetal effects (see below), perforated septum from "snorting," and HIV infection (from shared needles, if the drug is injected) are also deleterious consequences of cocaine abuse. Massive doses or bingeing on cocaine can result in respiratory paralysis, heart attacks (especially in men under forty years of age), convulsions and death.[3]

ABUSE OF AND DEPENDENCE ON COCAINE

Twenty-five years ago, cocaine was not believed to be an addicting drug because the discontinuation of chronic cocaine use did not produce typical physical withdrawal symptoms such as those observed with drugs like alcohol or heroin. It is now well known that cocaine is extremely addictive. Crack cocaine is also addictive. The euphoria produced by crack cocaine, for example, is so intense and the change in brain state so great, that craving for the drug develops after only a few trials.

Cocaine addiction (dependence) is not difficult to understand. Psychologically, cocaine is a potent mood elevator that produces (through changes in brain chemistry) unparalleled euphoria, exhilaration, and feelings of well-being and confidence. It increases alertness and decreases tension, self-doubt, and appetite. The laws of learning clearly predict that the elimination of an aversive state, coupled with a newfound euphoria, makes for a behavior likely to be repeated. Cocaine produces these effects by acting directly on pleasure centers in the brain such as the medial forebrain bundle (see Chapter 3).

Repeated use of cocaine results in insidious personality changes. Abusers become short-tempered, suspicious, and have difficulty concentrating. Cocaine abusers lose the ability to enjoy previously pleasurable activities, including sex. This state, called anhedonia, may last for many months. Schizoid behavior and personality changes may also develop. Frequent high doses of cocaine can result in cocaine psychosis. The drug-induced psychotic has delusions, paranoia, and may react violently against real or imagined persecution, which is similar to some forms of schizophrenia. Visual, tactile ("coke bugs"), and auditory hallucinations may last days, weeks, or months. Also, like psychotics, abusers have very little insight into their problem.

Some people use cocaine once or twice out of curiosity or some other reason and never use the drug again ("cocaine abusers"). Others seek treatment when their pattern of abuse and dependence leads to legal, financial, vocational, medical, psychological, or other problems. There is no single treatment for cocaine addiction. As with other drugs, overcoming denial of the problem and entering treatment are the first steps toward recovery. Some experts believe that cocaine is the most addicting drug of all.

COCAINE AND THE FETUS

Each year, between 91,500 and 240,000 neonates are exposed to cocaine through the mother's use of the drug.[4] When the mother uses cocaine, the drug's low molecular weight and high solubility enables it to pass freely through the placenta. The fetus is particularly sensitive to cocaine because, in contrast to the mature organism, low levels of fetal enzymes are unable to metabolize the drug and the fetus receives the full effect of the dose. This problem is made worse when the mother binges and high blood levels are obtained within minutes.

Cocaine acts as a vasoconstrictor in the mother as well as in the fetus, where it constricts blood vessels and decreases blood flow. This, in turn, decreases the blood oxygen supply to organs, and by the laws of physics, also increases blood pressure. In animal studies, fetal hypoxia is associated with growth retardation and congenital malformations. In humans, in-utero cocaine exposure coupled with other factors results in growth retardation, decreased head size, and increased risk for abruptio placentae, in which there is a premature separation of the placenta from the uterus, premature birth, and in some cases, death. Cocaine's effect on fetal heart rate and blood pressure may also contribute to cerebral hemorrhaging, infarctions, and other pregnancy complications. Unlike alcohol, cocaine-induced congenital malformations in humans are rare and not well documented. The term "fetal vascular disruption" has been offered to explain the array of observed cocaine-related malformations.

At birth, babies born of cocaine-abusing mothers are smaller in size, usually premature, require neonatal intensive care, have poor visual processing of faces and objects, abnormal sleep patterns, tremors, poor feeding, and transient central nervous system irritability. These findings should be interpreted cautiously since many of these effects may be due to concomitant use of alcohol, nicotine or other drugs, and poor nutrition. The long-term effects in these babies as they grow are not known.[5]

DOES COCAINE AFFECT DRIVING?

Laws against driving under the influence of alcohol usually include other drugs (e.g., cocaine). However, there are few controlled studies on the effects of cocaine on driving performance. At this time, a causative relationship between acute cocaine intoxication and driving accidents has not been established. On the other hand, behavioral effects of cocaine such as repetitive, focused, and impulsive actions are likely to impair the performance of complicated tasks such as driving an automobile.

AMPHETAMINE

Amphetamine and related compounds such as its derivative, methamphetamine (Methedrine), as well as dextroamphetamine (Dexedrine) and methylphenidate (Ritalin), are also potent stimulants, with biobehavioral actions similar to cocaine. Amphetamines exert their psychoactive effects for several hours longer than cocaine and they are somewhat less addicting and euphoric than cocaine.

Administration

1. *Oral:* The most common route of amphetamine administration.

2. *Insufflation:* Identical to cocaine. Rapid absorption into circulation through posterior nasal epithelium.

3. *Injection:* Highly water soluble. Intense rush in seconds.

Relatively low doses of amphetamine (e.g., 5 mg) produce an increased sense of well-being, decrease in fatigue and appetite, increased vigilance, and sympathomimetic effects, including increased heart rate, blood pressure, body temperature, and pupil dilation.

Neuropharmacology

Amphetamine exerts its biobehavioral effects by potentiating the release of brain dopamine, norepinephrine, and serotonin. Recent studies suggest that, as with cocaine, amphetamine also blocks the reuptake of dopamine.[6]

Half-Life

Amphetamine is eliminated primarily through excretion. As with most drugs that are eliminated through this route, the half-life varies considerably. In the case of amphetamines, the elimination half-life is about seven to thirty-four hours.

MEDICAL USES OF AMPHETAMINES

Amphetamine and amphetamine analogs such as Ritalin are effective in treating attention deficit hyperactivity disorders, presumably because of a feedback inhibition of overactive brain areas that mediate the symptoms of these disorders. However, attention deficit hyperactivity disorder (ADHD) may be caused by depression. Since amphetamine is also effective, to some degree, in alleviating depression, increasing attention and memory performance and learning in general, a child may more easily adjust to the environment if treated with amphetamine analogs such as Ritalin.

Although amphetamines are also used to treat narcolepsy (uncontrollable sleep episodes) and obesity, amphetamine use has been replaced by safer, more effective medications. Because of the abuse potential and other side effects of this drug, amphetamine is not the drug of choice.

ABUSE OF AND DEPENDENCE ON AMPHETAMINES

Chronic use of amphetamine produces a toxic psychosis or schizophrenia characterized by confused, disorganized behavior, stereotypy, paranoia, hallucinations, and delusions. Weight loss and skin ulcers (from injection infections) may also be observed in the chronic user.

Tolerance develops rapidly to the intoxicating effects of amphetamines but long-term chronic use is less common than binges or "runs" of several days.

Amphetamines are indeed highly addicting (dependence-producing). However, the opinion of those who treat Attention Deficit Disorder (ADD) is that giving ADD-diagnosed children amphetamines such as Dexedrine and Ritalin does not enhance the likelihood of addiction in those children.

XANTHINES

The last category of stimulants to be discussed rarely has serious biomedical or psychosocial consequences but is probably the most commonly used and therefore deserves some discussion. This category of stimulants is the xanthines, and includes caffeine, theophylline, and theobromine. These drugs are naturally derived from plants. Caffeine comes from coffee beans. Tea contains both caffeine and theophylline, and cocoa (as in chocolate) contains caffeine and theobromine. The nut of the cola tree also contains caffeine. Coca-Cola originally contained both cocaine (coca) and cola (caffeine) but cola drinks now contain only caffeine—about one-third the amount found in a cup of coffee for a typical serving.

Xanthines are almost always administered by oral absorption in beverages such as coffee or tea or in solid foods such as chocolate.

Caffeine is the most powerful of the xanthine stimulants. As with other stimulants, caffeine exerts sympathomimetic effects. The symptoms of caffeine intoxication include nervousness, diuresis, cardiac arrhythmias, rambling thoughts, insomnia, muscle twitching, or tremor. High doses can cause disorientation and a psychotic-like state, but this is rare.

Caffeine acts as a general cellular stimulant. The primary mechanism of action for caffeine involves the inhibition of phosphodiesterase, the enzyme that breaks down cAMP. Increasing available cAMP increases the phosphorylation of proteins in the membrane and changes the functional activity of the neuron (see Figure 7.2). Thus, caffeine acts, in part, on a second messenger system, but other as yet unidentified mechanisms may be involved.

Caffeine produces physical withdrawal (headache, gastrointestinal problems) and low-degree tolerance. But remember: tolerance and withdrawal are not sufficient to produce dependence (loss of control, addiction). Therefore, caffeine is generally not considered to be addicting under DSM-IV criteria.

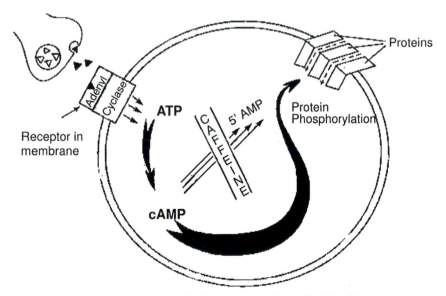

FIGURE 7.2. Neuropharmacological action of caffeine. Caffeine blocks the conversion of cAMP to 5'AMP, thereby increasing the activity of cAMP on protein kinase and ultimately the phosphorylation of proteins that alter the functional activity of the cell.

Chapter 8

Opioids:
Drugs That Calm Our Pain

*The prototype of these drugs is morphine, which has histori-
cally been used as a cure-all. Today, it is best known as a
powerful narcotic analgesic that is also highly addictive. It is
the prototype of a number of natural, synthetic, and semisynthetic opioids that have uses ranging from pain relief to cough
and diarrhea remedies. The study of opioids has provided
more pieces of the "puzzle" than any other area of psychopharmacology research. The most exciting fact about this
class of drugs is that they work through the excitation of brain
receptors that are also affected by naturally occurring opioids
called endorphins. These brain chemicals are probably
involved in determining our natural pain threshold, our exer-
cised-induced "high," and our response to addicting drugs. In
this chapter, we will explore the characteristics of different
types of opioids and how receptor antagonists (blockers) are
used both as antidotes to heroin overdose, and for the treatment of opiate addicts and alcohol-dependent patients.*

NATURAL OPIATES

Natural opiates (i.e., opium and codeine) come from the opium
poppy (*Papaver somniferum*), a vibrantly beautiful flowering plant
that blooms annually. The plants grow to a height of three or four
feet and have large flowers (4″ to 5″ in diameter) of various colors,
including white, pink, red, purple, or violet. The harvesting of raw

opium (see Figure 8.1) is an interesting process somewhat similar to the harvesting of maple sap. After the petals of the flower drop off, but before the large seed pod matures, the seed pod is scored (lightly cut). Overnight, a white substance appears, which, when it makes contact with the air, oxidizes to a gummy reddish brown resin. The resin is raw opium, which is scraped from the outside of the pod and can be smoked, eaten, or refined as desired.

The use of opiates goes back approximately 6,000 years. Opiates have been used as a cure-all for various diseases ranging from organic medical disorders to depression. Opiate use was widespread and opium was readily available for self-medication during the time of Hippocrates, the father of medicine (circa 470-370 B.C.). Opiates were a valuable commodity and as the opium trade grew, their use spread throughout Europe. Opium was generally considered a panacea for all human problems. As a narcotic analgesic, opium was

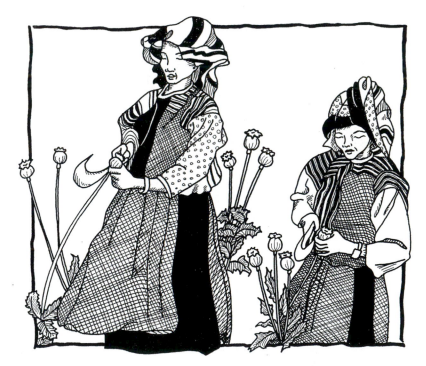

FIGURE 8.1. Harvesting of raw opium from the poppy plant *(Papaver somniferum).*

unsurpassed in its ability to decrease the response to pain, to suppress coughing, and to treat dysentery.

TERMINOLOGY

Opiates are drugs derived from opium and include morphine, codeine, and semisynthetic compounds derived from them, such as heroin. The term opioid is broader, including all agonists and antagonists with morphinelike activity, and including naturally occurring and synthetic opioid peptides, such as the endorphins.

Sometimes opioids are referred to as narcotics because they produce sleepiness or a dreamlike state also called a "nod" or stupor. Because of the Harrison Narcotic Act of 1914, which included marijuana as a narcotic, many legal statutes still use the term narcotic incorrectly—a problem that frequently occurs when people with legislative influence make decisions requiring scientific expertise!

USE AND POPULARITY

It was not until about 1806 that Frederich Sertürner, a German pharmacist, isolated the primary active ingredient in opium and named it morphium after the Greek god of dreams, Morphius. In 1832 codeine was similarly identified as the other psychoactive compound in opium. The identification of these compounds, coupled with the invention of the hypodermic syringe in the early 1850s, was enormously helpful in treating severe pain but increased the spread of addiction. Intravenous morphine was used regularly throughout the various wars of the nineteenth century including the American Civil War (1861-1865), the Prussian-Austrian War (1866), and the Franco-Prussian War (1870). Because the use of opiates was not regulated and they were available without prescription, returning veterans who had become addicted were able to maintain their addiction. Opiate addiction thus became known at the time as "soldier's disease."

During the nineteenth century, physicians were few and medical treatments were rather limited. To meet this need, a new industry emerged that promoted the use of various opiate-based tonics and elixirs, such as laudanum, a popular concoction of opium, wine, and various spices. These were inexpensive, socially acceptable, effective in relieving aches, pains, nervousness, diarrhea, and coughing, but they were nonetheless addictive because their primary active ingredients were opiates. Concern over the growing number of opiate addicts in the United States led to the development of the 1906 Food and Drugs Act and eventually the Harrison Narcotic Act, which mandated, among other things, a physician's prescription in order to obtain the drug.

SEMISYNTHETIC OPIATES

The widespread use, analgesic effectiveness, and potential for an ever-growing market led to additional research on the chemistry of opiates. In the late 1800s, it was found that adding two acetyl groups to the morphine molecule changed it to another compound, heroin. This new drug was introduced by Bayer Laboratories in 1898 as a nonaddicting pain reliever. The addition of the two acetyl groups to the morphine molecule significantly increased the drug's lipid solubility, enabling it to pass through the blood-brain barrier more rapidly. Once in the brain, heroin goes through a biotransformation and is converted back to morphine. The effects of heroin and morphine are identical, but heroin is about three times more potent and has a more rapid onset.

SYNTHETIC OPIOIDS

Methadone (Figure 8.2) is a synthetic opioid with a long half-life (eighteen to twenty-two hours). Methadone was developed during the Second World War by the Germans in response to decreased supplies of morphine and other anesthetics needed during wartime. Originally called Dolophine, after Adolf Hitler, methadone is frequently administered orally to treat heroin addicts. Methadone itself is addicting and psychoactive. However, when administered in a controlled clinical setting, it reduces the need to procure the drug on

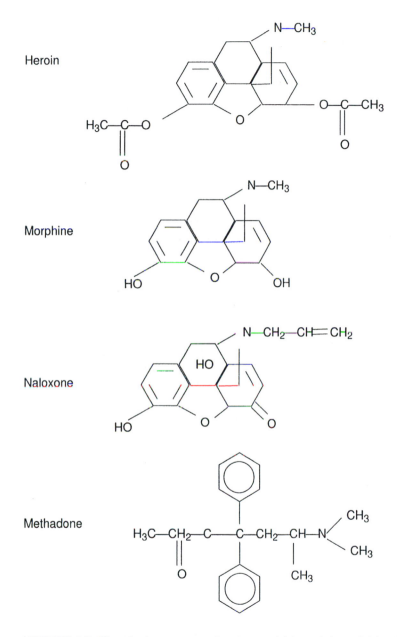

FIGURE 8.2. Chemical structures of various opioids and the opioid antagonist naloxone.

the street, in high doses will block the euphoria normally produced by heroin, eliminates risks associated with needle sharing (e.g., HIV, hepatitis), and allows the addict to engage in meaningful employment.

Meperidine (Demerol) is another synthetic opioid but with a much shorter half-life than methadone (see Table 8.1).

BRAIN OPIOID PEPTIDES

Why would the body respond to opioids at all? After all, these compounds are psychoactive, addictive, do not promote health, and can be toxic. In the early 1970s it was discovered that endogenous (from within) opiate receptors exist in the central nervous system. Subsequent studies have found opioid receptors in the gastrointestinal and other systems. Why would the body have such highly specific receptors?

The answer to this question is now obvious. The body itself must produce compounds that are very similar to exogenous opiates. The first two endogenous opioid peptides to be discovered were short-chained amino acid sequences named leucine-enkephalin and methionione-enkephalin. This discovery was soon followed by the discovery of a beta endorphin, a long thirty-one-amino-acid peptide whose first five amino acids were identical to methionione-enkephalin. It is now clear that various endorphins are manufactured within the brain and elsewhere, and act as part of the body's natural response to pain. For example, plasma endorphin levels increase during childbirth, traumatic accidents, and running. The latter may explain, in part, the "runner's high" frequently reported by athletes.

OPIOID ANTAGONISTS

Opioid antagonists are drugs that displace opiates and related compounds from their receptor sites. When these drugs are administered prophylactically, opiates are not able to produce intoxication. These antagonists are so effective in displacing opiates that they are effective in treating toxic overdoses. Naloxone (Narcan) is used for

TABLE 8.1. Pharmacological Characteristics of Common Opioids

Drug	Typical onset (min)	Peak effect (min)	Typical duration (hr)	Half-life (hr)	Equiv. Dose (mg) Intra-muscular	Equiv. Dose (mg) Oral	Source	Potency
Morphine	20	60	7	2-3	10	60	Natural	Strong
Heroin	15	60	4-5	—	—	—	Semisynthetic	Strong
Codeine	25	60	5	3-4	130	200	Natural	Intermediate
Meperidine (Demerol)	15	45	3	3-4	75	300	Synthetic	Strong
Dihydro-morphinone (Dilaudid)	25	60	5	3-4	1.5	8	Synthetic	Strong
Methadone (Dolophine)	15	120	5	22-25	10	20	Synthetic	Strong

Modified from Note 1. Values are approximations.

93

this purpose (Figure 8.2). Within seconds of intravenous administration, comatose patients with opioid overdoses rapidly regain consciousness. Naltrexone (ReVia, formerly Trexan) is a longer-acting antagonist used in the treatment of heroin and alcohol addicts.

ADMINISTRATION

1. *Oral:* The oldest route of opiate administration is oral. Opium cakes, candies, and various tonics containing the drug are traditional routes of administration. Because of the relatively low lipid solubility of naturally occurring opiates, oral administration is, although effective, not efficient in terms of maximum bioavailability. Methadone, a synthetic narcotic analgesic, is also administered orally.
2. *Pulmonary:* Interestingly, the widespread use of opium in China was tolerated well before the first millennium, but tobacco smoking was considered to be foul and offensive. By 1644 the Chinese emperor banned tobacco but not opium smoking in China. Because of the tobacco ban (which incidentally was very short-lived) opium smoking rapidly became a very popular method of administration.
3. *Insufflation:* Powdered opium and heroin can be insufflated ("snorted") and absorbed through the nasal membranes. Although opium is not well absorbed by this route, it is a frequently used method for first-time users. Heroin's high lipid solubility allows it to enter the circulation rapidly through insufflation.
4. *Injection:* Morphine, which is available as a liquid, or other water soluble narcotics (such as heroin), can be injected using all three injection sites: intravenous, intramuscular, and subcutaneous.

DISTRIBUTION AND ELIMINATION

All opioids are distributed throughout the body, including the central nervous system where they exert their psychoactive effects. Natural opiates, because of their relatively low lipid solubility, gen-

TABLE 8.2. Biobehavioral Effects of Opioids

- constricted pupils (miosis)
- decreased pulse
- decreased temperature
- decreased respiration
- slowed reflexes
- slow, low, raspy, slurred speech
- skin cool to the touch
- nausea (new users)
- impaired memory and attention
- stupor or coma (overdose)

erally do not enter the brain as quickly as semisynthetic opioids such as heroin. As with other drugs, if the opioid is smoked it enters the circulation almost immediately, with high blood levels occurring within minutes.

Opiates are metabolized by the liver. The half-life of most opioids is relatively short, approximately three hours. The one major exception to this is methadone, which has a prolonged plasma half-life (see Table 8.1).

MEDICAL USES

The primary use of opioid analgesics such as morphine is in the treatment of pain. Opioids are extremely effective in reducing the affective ("suffering") component of pain. When under the influence of these drugs, people know the pain is there but do not respond to it. Opioids, usually in the form of codeine, are very effective in treating coughs, although synthetic derivatives such as dextromethorphan are also effective without the sedating and addicting properties.

HARMFUL EFFECTS: MYTHS AND REALITIES

In comparison to many other psychoactive drugs, opioids have relatively few medical consequences. That does not mean that opioid analgesics are safe! They have a high potential for addiction and overdose. Opioids decrease the activity of those brainstem regions that monitor blood CO_2. Death by respiratory depression is the usual consequence of an opioid overdose. Most opioids stimulate those neurons in the medulla that are part of the vomit reflex. As a result, users experience nausea from drugs such as heroin until they develop tolerance.

Opioids and the Fetus

Pregnant women who are addicted to heroin place their fetuses at risk should they go through withdrawal or when they give birth, because the abrupt termination of the drug to the child may be very uncomfortable. Children born of heroin-addicted mothers are restless, irritable, and tremulous, and have a high-pitched cry, gooseflesh, runny nose, and other adultlike withdrawal symptoms.

Pregnant women who are addicted to heroin give birth to infants that are smaller in overall size and head circumference than control subjects of mothers not using heroin. Methadone, a synthetic opioid used to treat heroin addicts, is a relatively safe alternative to heroin, but it is still an addictive drug. Compared to control subjects (children whose mothers did not take methadone), methadone-exposed infants have poorer fine and gross motor coordination at birth. By age five, these children are more active, engage in task-irrelevant activity, and have poorer fine-motor coordination than controls. There are conflicting reports regarding the effects of prenatal opioid exposure on cognitive development in toddlers and preschoolers. Observations of delayed mental and motor development may be due to poor environmental conditions, or methadone may produce subtle neurological changes, making children more susceptible to the developmental delays associated with impoverished environments. Mothers who use heroin often use other drugs (nicotine, etc.) and are poorly nourished with poor prenatal care. Thus, many factors may contribute to fetal distress after birth.

ABUSE OF AND DEPENDENCE ON OPIOIDS

Tolerance to opiates develops within only a few days of use and increases throughout the addiction process. Tolerance to opioids is often quite remarkable. In some cases, there may be little or no observed impairment in the intoxicated addict. Tolerance develops to the euphoric and analgesic effects of analgesics as well as to some of the side effects (nausea). Tolerance does not develop to the effects of these narcotic analgesics on pupil constriction and only slight tolerance develops to their constipating effects. Among chronic addicts, even high doses of the drug will produce little pleasurable effect and the drug is taken primarily to avoid the consequences of withdrawal.

Opioids, regardless of their origin (natural, semisynthetic, synthetic), produce physical dependence. The regular use of these drugs produces withdrawal symptoms upon cessation of use. Withdrawal from narcotic analgesics is very rarely life-threatening. The symptoms of withdrawal are similar to a very severe bout of influenza. Addicts feel achy, weak, irritable, hypersensitive, and have a runny nose. Some of these symptoms begin within a few hours of the last drug use. Maximum withdrawal symptoms, which include a spastic jerky movement ("kicking the habit"), occur about forty-eight to seventy-two hours after the last dose.

Interestingly, there is a great deal of clinical interest in detoxification of opioid addicts, in spite of the generally-held belief that withdrawal from opioids does not enhance abstinence outcome. However, there are several methods for detoxification.

- "Cold Turkey"—patient abstains and goes through withdrawal without any special treatment. Withdrawal in this manner is very uncomfortable but not lethal.

- Medicated Withdrawal

    Clonidine (Catapres) reduces the uncomfortable nervous system hyperexcitability associated with withdrawal. Another drug, lofexidine, has also been used in this way but is still considered experimental.

    Phenobarbital reduces overall withdrawal symptoms.

- Alternative Treatments

    Acupuncture is also effective in reducing withdrawal severity in some patients.

After detoxification, long-term treatment of opioid dependence follows one of two philosophies: total abstinence or assisted abstinence. To achieve abstinence, opioid addicts are encouraged to attend therapeutic centers or communities to learn how to live drug-free. Aids to abstinence include naltrexone (ReVia), an opioid antagonist that blocks the euphoric effects of opioids; and buprenorphine (Buprenex), an opioid agonist/antagonist that has been suggested to reduce the craving for other opioids such as heroin. Some opioid addicts are able to become permanently abstinent from all addictive drugs through these programs.

The best methadone programs are those in which the patient is required to take the medication in the clinic, urine screens are required to monitor other drug use, and patients are required to maintain an outside job and attend therapy or twelve-step (Narcotics Anonymous) sessions. LAAM, a long-acting methadone that does not have to be given every day, is also available to use in these programs. The intent is to wean an addict off the opioid drug (usually heroin); but many addicts are maintained on methadone for the rest of their lives, because they cannot or do not commit to abstinence. "Effectiveness" of treatment in such programs is therefore not measured by an abstinence outcome, but by the quality of life achieved by the opioid-addicted patient.

Unlike most other psychoactive and abused drugs, chronic opiate abuse is not generally associated with liver, heart, brain, or other organ damage.

Opiates are highly addicting, meaning that they create a strong "need" in the opiate-dependent individual. This dependence is very difficult to break, which can lead to lifelong opiate use. Complicating the picture is the fact that addicts know that opiates are relatively organ-nontoxic, so they see little harm in continuing to use them. This is the reason that methadone is such a controversial treatment: Opiate addicts often use methadone (or more powerful opiate agonists) for the rest of their lives. Yet the abstinence concept of treatment conflicts with this outcome.

Chapter 9

Marijuana:
The Illegal Recreational Plant

This interesting drug has reached a level of controversy in social discussions that is unmatched in the history of our nation, except for the last time someone suggested legalizing drugs. Marijuana is addicting, yet it has no known lethal dose in humans, is far less toxic to humans than alcohol or nicotine, and is even used (legally, in some states) as a treatment for AIDS and cancer patients. Anecdotal evidence suggests that it is truly recreational in low to moderate amounts, yet in higher amounts it definitely causes lack of motivation, short-term memory loss, and impairs driving skills when a person is intoxicated. The best we can say about this drug is that the only answer to its controversial consequences is that more scientific research is needed. Let's examine some facts and myths about this drug.

WHAT IS MARIJUANA?

Throughout history plants have provided humans with a variety of uses. In addition to being a source of food, fiber, shelter, herbal and other medicines, and oxygen, some are consumed because they contain psychoactive compounds. One such plant is cannabis. In this country, the term "marijuana" is used to describe the whole plant or any part of it. A typical plant is illustrated in Figure 9.1. The leaves are always variegated (of various shapes) but may be long and thin or short and elliptical depending upon the species. Some varieties, such as *Cannabis indicia,* rarely grow more than

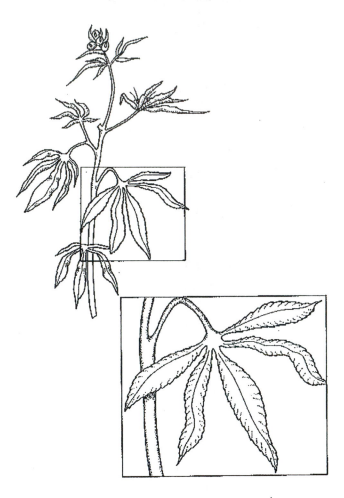

FIGURE 9.1. Cannabis plant.

four to five feet tall, whereas *Cannabis sativa* can reach heights of fifteen feet or more.

Cannabis probably originated in the Orient, but different species grow wild or are cultivated for various uses in many different regions of the world. In fact, George Washington grew *Cannabis sativa* on his farm in Mount Vernon, probably to make hemp rope.

Since the weed grows well in moderate climates, it spreads readily and is now wild throughout many portions of the United States. Today, marijuana horticulture is estimated at $32 billion per year, making it one of the largest cash crops in America.

WHAT IS THC?

Cannabis contains a psychoactive substance called delta-9-tetra-hydrocannabinol (THC). Most illicit use of cannabis is related to the psychoactive effects of THC. One species of the plant, *Cannabis indicia*, has a relatively high concentration of THC, harsh taste, is quite hearty, and will grow in most areas where other weeds can survive. The other major species, *Cannabis sativa*, has relatively low concentrations of THC, a smooth taste, and does not grow well in colder climates. Marijuana cultivators have experimented with hybrids to obtain the best of both species. The cultivation, showing, and sale of this plant have become a cult-like cottage industry in recent years. In general, the concentration of THC in street-purchased marijuana has increased from about 0.5 to 2 percent in the 1970s to as high as about 10 percent in the 1990s.

THC is found in the saplike resin of the cannabis plant (Figure 9.2). The greatest concentration of THC is found in the flowering tops of the plant, with less in the leaf and stalk. This drug can be prepared in different ways depending upon the part of the plant used. For example, in India, charas is made from a pure form of the resin, which is carefully removed from the flower, leaf, and plant stem. Sinsemilla comes from the seedless bud of the female plant and ganja is made from the dried flower tops of the female plant. Bhang is prepared from the dried leaf and stem powder and is usually served in a drink or as candy.

HOW IS MARIJUANA ADMINISTERED?

The most common route of administration is through the pulmonary system, although the plant can be ingested and absorbed through the gastrointestinal system as well. Most marijuana is milled and smoked

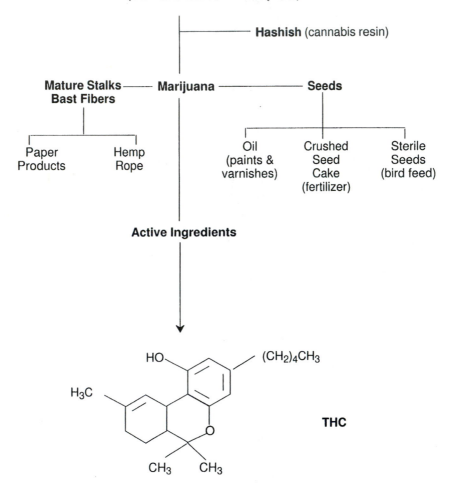

FIGURE 9.2. The cannabis plant is used in the manufacture of many legal products. Illegal compounds such as delta-9-tetrahydrocannabinol (shown) or cannabidiol are primarily responsible for the psychoactive effects of marijuana and hashish, respectively. (Adapted from Phillips, 1985.)[1]

like tobacco in a pipe or in hand-rolled cigarettes often called "joints" or "bones," because of their appearance. Usually, the dried plant leaf is smoked. The stem and seeds may also be smoked, but they are not nearly as potent as the leaf. When smoked, THC enters the circulation as an airborne particle and is rapidly distributed into the blood. The blood carries THC to various tissues, including the brain. Definite effects are noticeable to the smoker within several minutes. THC may be taken orally as well (in brownies, for example); however, the amount of drug required to produce psychoactive effects is approximately two to three times more than when it is smoked. This difference is probably due to bioavailability. More drug enters the blood through the lungs than through the gastrointestinal tract.

DISTRIBUTION

When smoked, THC enters the circulation almost immediately, reaching very high blood levels within five to ten minutes. Although the psychoactive effects begin within minutes, the relationship between reports of being "highest" and peak blood level is not as highly correlated as for some other drugs. The greatest subjective high usually occurs after peak concentrations in blood are reached; in some studies, this occurs roughly fifteen to forty-five minutes after smoking. One explanation for this might be that the high is produced by a combination of THC and one of its active metabolites. Since the metabolite 11-hydroxy-delta-9-THC has effects nearly identical to the parent compound, it is possible that both compounds combine in an additive fashion. Thus, it may take some additional time after peak THC levels in blood for metabolites to form and the subjective high to be reached. However, empirical evidence to support this notion is lacking. There are fairly large differences among (1) how individuals feel, (2) drug potency, and (3) average doses. The high from a single joint usually lasts up to about two hours, but residual effects can last much longer.

DIFFERENT TYPES OF MARIJUANA

There are different species of the cannabis plant, including hybrids designed to have high THC content. Marijuana is called many different names depending on geographical and cultural factors. A few of its other names are: grass, Maryjane, pot, MJ, Jane, smoke, weed, boo, reefer, dope, doobie, and tea. Often marijuana comes in different colors (e.g., gold, red, black, greenish-brown). "Acapulco" or "Colombian gold" is produced by shearing the roots on one side of the plant with a shovel a few days before harvest. This cuts off about half of the roots and interrupts the supply of plant hormones that prevent discoloration. By interrupting the supply of plant hormone, chlorophyll breaks down and the plant takes on a golden color. "Punta Roja" appears red naturally, whereas "African Wacky" appears black because the cells of the harvested plant are squashed (the plant is run through the rollers of an old-fashioned wringer washing machine or similar device) and left to ferment like black tea. The most common marijuana color is greenish-brown, but color has little to do with actual potency, despite marketing efforts to convince buyers otherwise. Some hybrids, such as Potomac Indica or Northern Lights, do have high THC content and are very potent. The plant components that make up marijuana vary considerably, but generally the entire plant is milled like tobacco and smoked. Some users will only smoke the unpollinated bud of the female plant (Sinsemilla); the remainder of the plant (called "shake") is considered not worth smoking.

Hashish, like charas, is relatively pure and is made by scraping the resin from the plant. Hashish also comes in different colors and textures. These range from golden blocks that crumble into fine powder, to dark, dense, oily blocks. Hashish is usually smoked in a small pipe, but it is occasionally eaten (e.g., "hash" brownies or cookies).

Marijuana is sold in kilograms (about 2.2 pounds) but more commonly in ounces, grams, or individual "joints." Hashish is also sold in chunks that are fractions of an ounce or kilogram.

WHO USES MARIJUANA?

Cannabis has always had a certain mystery associated with its use. Part of the intrigue comes from legends from the Mediterranean area about the use of hashish by a religious cult called the Hashishiyya. The Hashishiyya murdered political enemies for their leader, Hasan-Ibn-Sabbah, from whose name the term assassin is probably derived. By the middle of the 1800s, the use of hashish had spread through Europe and appears in such literary works as *The Count of Monte Cristo* (Dumas), *Le Club Hachischins* (Gautier) and *Artificial Paradise* (Baudelaire). The descriptions of hashish intoxication found in these works are quite accurate and make for very interesting reading.

The use of marijuana and hashish increased dramatically during the 1950s and 1960s when a large portion of our society "turned on, tuned in and dropped out." As public interest and concern grew, social scientists began monitoring drug use through detailed, anonymous questionnaire surveys. The target population for many of these studies was high school students. Based on the results of large scale, nationally distributed surveys, it appears that regular use of this drug was quite common. However, during the period 1980-1994, there was a decline in marijuana use in the United States. The reason for this change is not known; however, one factor may be student attitudes about the risks associated with it. Increased awareness about the health risks of smoking, in general, as well as increased awareness about drugs may have contributed to this change in attitude. However, for a number of reasons, marijuana use by high school students rose again in 1995-1996.

Another factor that influences use is availability. Improved law enforcement techniques make successful smuggling of this bulky product hazardous. As a result, drug traffickers are now concentrating on importing more easily concealed drugs, such as cocaine, which ultimately yields a greater profit. Again, as a result of supply and demand, the use of homegrown marijuana is increasing in many areas. Thus, marijuana use is still very widespread. In 1995, for example, 42 percent of all high school students had tried marijuana, over 20 percent of all high school seniors reported that they smoked marijuana monthly, and 5 percent reported daily use.[2]

NEUROPHARMACOLOGY OF CANNABINOIDS

There are more than 400 different chemicals in the marijuana plant including about 60 compounds called cannabinoids. These are the pharmacologically active substances in marijuana and other products of the cannabis plant. There are four major cannabinoids, of which the most psychoactive is delta-9-tetrahydrocannabinol

(Δ-9-THC), whose structure is illustrated at the bottom of Figure 9.2. In hashish, the primary psychoactive compound is a structurally related compound, cannabidiol (CBD). In addition to Δ-9-THC, metabolites or breakdown products of this compound, such as 11-hydroxy-Δ-9 THC, are also psychoactive. Thus, unlike many drugs, the metabolism of Δ-9-THC by liver enzymes does not decrease intoxication, it prolongs it.

Given the range of marijuana's biobehavioral effects, it should not be surprising to learn that molecular receptors for cannabis are distributed most densely throughout the cerebellum, basal ganglia, and hippocampus of the brain. These areas allow movement, emotions, and memory. THC inhibits the activity of adenyl cyclase, an enzyme that stimulates cAMP to alter the excitability of the neuron. The greater the psychoactive effect of the drug, the greater the inhibition of the enzyme.[3]

Interestingly, there are about a hundred times as many marijuana receptors as opiate receptors in the brain. One might wonder why the brain has so many receptors for this drug. The answer should be obvious—the brain must manufacture an endogenous compound with properties similar to THC. The brain does in fact contain a naturally present molecule called anandamide that binds to the marijuana receptors. Current research is designed to determine whether anandamide mimics all the actions of cannabis at its receptor in the brain.

HALF-LIFE AND MEASUREMENT OF THC

THC has a half-life of about twenty-four hours, so most of the drug is completely out of the blood within a week. THC metabolites can be detected for as many as forty-five to sixty days after the last use, depending upon the method of analysis. Because THC and its metabolites are highly fat soluble, these compounds are stored in, and slowly released from, fat tissue. This has two implications: the first is that by analyzing a sample of blood or urine, it is easy to determine whether or not someone has used marijuana in the last month or two. Second, the test alone does not provide bona fide evidence that the person was intoxicated at the time of testing (see below). Behavioral evidence of intoxication or other indications of recent use are needed for such a conclusion. Marijuana can be detected in most body fluids, including serum, blood, saliva, or urine, using a variety of analytical methods, including thin layer chromatography (TLC), high pressure liquid chromatography (HPLC), gas chromatography (GC), gas chromatography/mass spectrometry (GC/MS), enzyme immunoassay (EIA), and radioimmunoassay (RIA).

These laboratory tests are used to detect THC compounds. The ones that are extremely sensitive are also very expensive to run. The EMIT test of urine (an EIA), is sensitive down to 25 nanograms per milliliter (ng/ml). TLC and RIA are capable of detecting THC or its metabolites in the 1-5 ng/ml range and GC/MS can detect as little as 0.5-1 ng/ml. Since 1 nanogram is equal to 1/1,000,000,000th of a gram and 1 ml (milliliter) is equal to about 1/30 of a fluid ounce, you can see that these tests are extremely sensitive. Smoking two joints, one every two hours, will raise plasma Δ-9-THC in the blood to roughly 40-50 ng/ml within ten minutes. Yet six hours after the second joint, Δ-9-THC levels are still around 5 ng/ml. THC metabolites can be detected in urine weeks or months after the last dose.[4]

While these tests are accurate and obviously quite sensitive, they may not be quantitative. In many cases, laboratories detect THC through the presence of metabolites only. Since not all metabolites are psychoactive, a "positive for THC" test in body fluids does not necessarily provide scientific information about (1) how much was administered, (2) when the drug was taken, or (3) the effect of the drug on behavior or physiology. Most forensic urine tests for THC measure the major metabolite 11-nor-9-carboxy-Δ-9-THC (9-carboxy-THC), which itself is not psychoactive. In fact, there is some concern that with extremely sensitive test procedures, people who passively inhale marijuana smoke or who are exposed to other forms of involuntary consumption of THC would test positive for the drug. Studies on passive inhalation or absorption through the skin (from handling marijuana) have not been conclusive.

BIOBEHAVIORAL EFFECTS
AND USE OF MARIJUANA

The psychoactive properties of cannabis have been known for nearly 5,000 years, with the earliest reference dating back to the

Shen Nung dynasty in China, circa 2737 B.C. Cannabis was taken to treat a wide range of ailments including "female weakness," rheumatism, malaria, beriberi, constipation, and absent-mindedness. When mixed with wine it was used as an anesthetic. By the year 1000 A.D. cannabis had reached northern Africa, where its reputation and use flourished.

The most common legal use of cannabis is for the manufacture of rope and birdseed. (The cannabis seeds used in birdseed contain very little THC.) The active ingredient in cannabis has been used to treat certain medical ailments such as glaucoma (increased pressure in the eye), and to treat some of the side effects (e.g., nausea) associated with cancer chemotherapy. Some of the more common products of the cannabis plant are shown in Figure 9.2.

General Effects

Marijuana users describe the effects of the drug along different dimensions. Not all effects are experienced simultaneously, or in every user each time they administer the drug. Some of the more consistently reported effects are described in Table 9.1.[5]

Most people who smoke marijuana believe that marijuana enhances pleasurable things even more. Users report that sex is much more physically enjoyable because of enhanced tactile sensations. This effect has been offered as evidence that marijuana use

TABLE 9.1: Common Subjective Effects of Marijuana Intoxication

- Relaxed
- Thirsty
- Touch/sensations enhanced
- Metaphysical thoughts/euphoric
- Time distortion (sense that time slows down)
- Metaphysical thoughts (often perceived as very profound)
- Euphoria
- Food tastes/cravings enhanced ("munchies")
- Dry (cotton) mouth
- Colors look more vibrant
- Bouts of spontaneous laughter—common events seem funny
- Memory impairment (especially short term)

- decreased risk-taking.

increases promiscuity in women or rape in men, but the scientific evidence that there is a causal relationship is slim. At best, it may suggest that people who use marijuana are part of a subculture that has more liberal attitudes toward sex. There is no scientific evidence that marijuana leads to rape. (Rape is thought to be a crime of violence, not a crime of passion). In contrast, use of marijuana is usually associated with feelings of relaxation and decreased tension, not violence.

After smoking a joint, most marijuana users report dry ("cotton") mouth and an increase in appetite, especially for snack foods. Interestingly, the "munchies" are not associated with changes in blood glucose, which normally stimulate hunger.

Marijuana has so many pharmacological and biobehavioral actions that it is classified separately from other drugs. The drug is sometimes described as a hallucinogen; however, it rarely produces frank hallucinations, except at extremely high doses. Marijuana users tend to consume low doses of the drug so that they do not experience hallucinations, although differences in tolerance, experience, and drug potency may lead to unexpected and undesired toxic effects.

Medical Uses

THC does have some potential medical uses. As a bronchodilator, THC may be useful in the treatment of asthma, particularly when other medications are not effective. However, under such circumstances, the drug would probably best be administered orally, rather than through the pulmonary system, since particles in smoke would irritate sensitive lung tissue and exacerbate the asthma. Long-term use of THC as an antiasthmatic may be contraindicated since there is also evidence that chronic use of marijuana results in bronchoconstriction.

THC is also effective in treating glaucoma, but other antiglaucoma drugs are available, so this medical use of THC is not approved by the Drug Enforcement Administration (DEA). Glaucoma is a disease characterized by increased intraocular pressure and is the second leading cause of blindness in the United States. Eventually, the pressure within the eyeball increases to the point that the optic nerve, which sends information from the eye to the brain, is damaged. Clinical case studies suggest that marijuana may cause a dose-dependent decrease in intraocular pressure, lasting for several hours. Although the use of marijuana will not cure glaucoma, it can slow down the progressive loss of vision. Inhalation, oral consumption, or intravenous injection of THC are about equally effective in treating glaucoma, whereas topical administration (e.g., eye drops) is not. The psychoactive effects associated with THC treatment may not be well tolerated by some patients.

Perhaps the most accepted medical use of THC is with cancer patients. Dronabinol, a THC drug, has been found to be very effective in controlling the severe nausea and vomiting associated with chemotherapy. Dronabinol (Marinol) is a Schedule II THC drug. It can only be obtained by prescription through physicians registered with the National Cancer Institute and the DEA. In addition to using THC in the treatment of these conditions, the National Academy of Sciences concluded that THC/marijuana might also be useful in treating seizures, spasticity, and other nervous system disorders.

Recently, some states have voted to allow physicians to recommend marijuana for medical use, particularly for AIDS patients, terminally-ill cancer patients, and people in severe pain. While there is insufficient research evidence for some of these therapeutic benefits, the controlled use of marijuana for patients with few other options constitutes a valid benefit-risk decision by physicians.

HARMFUL EFFECTS: MYTHS AND REALITIES

Communication, Memory, Driving, and Motivation

Many undesirable side effects are associated with marijuana use. The most common is the false sense of enhanced creativity and ability to communicate. In a social environment where the perception of enhanced abilities may have few significant consequences, such effects are relatively benign. However, in a working or learning environment where the decisions made by an intoxicated person or the actual quality of their material work may affect the individual or group, such effects may be quite harmful.

Short-term memory is greatly impaired by marijuana use. This may result in a deterioration of goal-directed behavior, particularly when the user must go through several steps to successfully complete a task. In a social setting, a short-term memory lapse that leads you to forget what you were about to do or say may appear quite humorous and may actually be part of the desired high. At the workplace, at home, in school, or elsewhere, such psychoactive effects are obviously harmful. In other situations, such as driving a motor vehicle, these effects may be dangerous.

Most field research on motor vehicle accidents makes it difficult to single out marijuana intoxication as the cause of an accident, because most of the drivers were drinking alcohol as well. Therefore, alcohol intoxication may have been listed as the only cause of the accident. Controlled field studies also indicate that marijuana decreases risk-taking while driving (e.g., fewer unsafe passes, decreased speed). However, the contribution of marijuana intoxication cannot be ignored when one considers how important memory is to safe driving and that marijuana impairs memory. Consider the following, for example. To safely exit from a highway requires several steps, including remembering what exit you want, remaining vigilant for the exit, signaling your intention to change lanes, checking your mirror and blind spots for other cars, executing a lane change and slowing down to exit ramp speed. Forgetting to do any of these steps can result in an accident.

In a controlled study, subjects driving experimental vehicles while under the influence of marijuana responded fairly well to emergency situations when they were given advance notice that they must respond. However, when there was no warning of the emergency response, subjects under the influence of marijuana were impaired in their ability to make emergency decisions.

Strength, Coordination, and Judgment

In the laboratory, very low doses of THC have been shown to have little effect on the performance of motor tasks and reaction time. However, at commonly used doses, THC has profound deleterious effects. Laboratory studies have shown that the ability to drive a car or fly an airplane is seriously impaired by one to two joints due to decreases in muscular strength, coordination, judgment, and perception of time and distance. Of particular concern is that this impairment lasts four to eight hours—well past the subjective high produced by the drug.[6,7] The user feels unimpaired several hours after the peak effects; however, the drug continues to produce impairment when measured objectively. Field studies of marijuana's effects on driving are difficult to interpret because in most cases other drugs (e.g., alcohol) are present in such high concentrations that they could account for any effects on driving.

There have been many reports that chronic marijuana use leads to apathy and loss of interest in accomplishments, slow thinking, and other cognitive impairments. Unfortunately, these reports failed to determine whether such cognitive impairments existed prior to chronic marijuana use or were directly related to the use of the drug. Objective scientific evidence for "amotivational syndrome" produced by chronic marijuana use is still lacking. Even so, marijuana intoxication impairs basic cognitive processes such as memory and distorts perception. To the extent that these are the foundations of learning and motivation, chronic marijuana use is harmful. Poor learning usually results in poor performance, and poor performance can be a disincentive to future learning. Thus, a cascading loop of failure can develop. Additional research is needed to study the effects of long-term moderate and heavy use of this drug on psychological and physiological processes.

Marijuana and Crime

At about the same time as the alcohol prohibition movement started gaining momentum in the United States, newspaper articles linking marijuana use to violent crime attracted public interest and concern. Even though the link between marijuana use and violence stemmed from a few isolated incidents and there was no concrete evidence that marijuana caused violence, by 1936 most states had laws regulating the use, sale, and possession of cannabis. These regulations coupled with a very high tax on growers, distributors, and buyers made legal use of cannabis almost impossible. In 1969 the U.S. Supreme Court declared that a marijuana "tax law" was unconstitutional because it violated the Fifth Amendment. Since this constitutional amendment protects people from self-incrimination, declaring marijuana use on your tax return would be in violation of a constitutional right and of the Fifth Amendment.

Despite major legislation aimed at preventing the use of marijuana and considerable speculation about its harmful effects, there had been little scientific research on the drug up through the 1930s and 1940s. To determine what course of legal action should be taken to protect the public from the consequences of marijuana use, New York City Mayor Fiorello LaGuardia asked the New York academy of Medicine to look into the matter. The academy issued a report in 1944 in which they concluded that the acute use of marijuana impaired intellectual functioning but did not alter the basic personality of users, nor did chronic use produce mental or physical deterioration.[8] Although this report met with violent criticism from the American Medical Association, the LaGuardia Report agrees with previous studies as well as subsequent ones.

Marijuana intoxication impairs many cognitive functions, including judgment, which can lead to poor decisions regarding present behavior and future outcomes, for example. However, there is little scientific evidence that marijuana use is associated with an increase in violent or aggressive behavior.

Cardiovascular System

One of the most consistent effects of acute marijuana intoxication is increased heart rate or tachycardia. A normal resting heart rate is about 70 to 90 beats per minute. During intoxication, tachycardia of twenty to fifty beats per minute above normal is average. A heart rate of 140 beats per minute is not uncommon. The effects of marijuana on blood pressure are variable. For example, there is evidence that while intoxicated, blood pressure is increased while lying down, but decreased when standing.

Panic Attacks

Although less often reported, anxiety, depression, and paranoia may occur, usually following high doses of THC. The incidence of these is quite low, but may be more common among less experienced marijuana users. Regardless of experience, panic attacks can be quite serious. Should such a reaction occur, get the person to a hospital emergency room. The following treatment guidelines may be helpful.

First, determine if other intoxicating drugs or preexisting medical disorders are contributing to the symptoms. This can be accomplished through oral report of the user, witnesses, and/or a blood or urine drug screen.

Second, the patient should be assured that "it is only a drug" and the symptoms will stop in less than five to eight hours. Decreasing outside stimulation by placing the patient in a quiet room and "talking them down" is also helpful. Generally, the use of other drugs to treat a panic attack is not recommended unless the reaction is uncontrollable. Under such circumstances, an anxiolytic such as alprazolam (Xanax), 6 mg daily, can be prescribed.

Finally, patients should be warned that metabolites of the drug will remain in the body for several days and that they may experience mild drug effects during that time, but that the effects are not permanent.

Brain Damage

Ultimately, the effects of marijuana on behavior are mediated by changes in the central nervous system. Considerable attention has been given to studies that purport to demonstrate brain damage following marijuana use. The first wave of such studies, conducted during the early 1970s, suggested that marijuana produced atrophy of the cerebral cortex (as reflected by enlarged ventricles within the brain). Critical reviews of such studies revealed that in addition to smoking marijuana, many of the subjects had head injuries, epilepsy, and poly-drug use histories. Thus, the conclusion that marijuana produces cerebral atrophy, even among heavy users, was unjustified. More recent studies using computerized tomography (CAT scans) have produced conflicting results.

Central nervous system dysfunction and gross neuropathology may also be assessed using an electroencephalogram (EEG). For the most part, acute cannabis intoxication enhances brain alpha wave activity and decreases beta wave activity. However, these acute effects are not cannabis-specific, or surprising, as they occur with many sedative drugs. Moreover, it should be kept in mind that EEG changes occur constantly in the normal, drug-free brain. Non-drug studies have suggested that alpha activity is associated with a relaxed mental state whereas beta activity is associated with problem solving and other mental activities. Although some studies have demonstrated that THC can produce specific changes in the electrical activity of specific brain cells in animals, the relationship between such changes and behavior (in animals or humans) remains to be determined.

Cancer

Of great concern is the increasing scientific literature indicating that the combustion of marijuana, like tobacco leaf, produces tars and other products that increase the risk of lung cancer. For many years, advocates of marijuana use suggested that it was less harmful to smoke marijuana than it was to smoke cigarettes. That no longer seems to be true. Although heavy users probably smoke fewer marijuana cigarettes than the average heavy tobacco user smokes, a typical joint contains two to three times the amount of tar found in some popular brands of cigarettes. Coupled with the fact that, like many cigarette smokers, marijuana smokers inhale deeply and hold the smoke to maximize the intake of the drug, the risk of pulmonary hazards as well as lung cancer is sufficiently strong to warrant concern among chronic marijuana users.

Immune System

The immune system is made up of specialized cells (lymphocytes) that protect us from invading infectious or allergic diseases. By quickly responding to invading antigens, the body's immune system can combat many illnesses. There is some evidence that chronic marijuana use decreases the functioning of the immune system when measured strictly in terms of immunological response. However, it is not known whether such changes have any clinical significance. In other words, marijuana seems to impair the immune system in scientific studies, but there is little evidence that this leads to increased susceptibility to illness or disease.

Sex Hormones

Marijuana use reduces testosterone, the male sex hormone responsible for the development of secondary sexual characteristics and sperm cell production. Researchers have found that in humans, after four to six weeks of daily use, testosterone levels are depressed but still within normal limits. There is evidence that THC temporarily decreases levels of luteinizing hormone, a reproductive hormone in females. The clinical significance of this effect or the effect of chronic THC use in humans requires further study.

Toxicity

THC, in comparison to other psychoactive drugs, does not seem to be very lethal. In experimental studies, dogs given extremely high doses of THC have not died. Statistical projections from animal data to humans suggests that there is about a 20,000-fold difference between therapeutic doses of THC and the lethal dose. Although such projections are only estimates, there are no known cases of a lethal overdose in humans from smoking marijuana.

MARIJUANA AND THE FETUS

It is difficult to measure marijuana effects on the fetus, because few women use only marijuana during pregnancy. More often, other variables such as alcohol, smoking cigarettes, and poor prenatal care produce an unclear picture. Nevertheless, evidence is accumulating that the use of marijuana during pregnancy may increase risk for premature birth, small birth size, and delayed development. To date, most studies reveal no clear relationship between maternal marijuana use and physical birth defects in humans, although some defects have been reported, such as craniofacial features similar to FAS. At birth, marijuana-exposed infants tend to have poorer habituation to visual stimuli, fine tremors, and increased startle responses to spontaneous and mild stimuli. However, at twelve months of age, mental, visual, and motor performance are not significantly correlated with maternal use of marijuana. More subtle, long-term effects have not yet been seen.

There is some evidence that marijuana use causes chromosomal damage in some cells. Chromosomes are components within the nucleus of cells that carry the genetic information unique to each individual and necessary for cell replication and reproduction. There is also evidence that marijuana does *not* affect chromosomes. Even though the mechanism of marijuana's effects on the fetus have not yet been identified, the safe public health message is that marijuana use during pregnancy should be avoided. Moreover, high concentrations of THC are also secreted into the milk of nursing mothers, probably because of the high fat content of milk. Hence, the use of marijuana during nursing should also be avoided.

Finally, since marijuana impairs memory and other cognitive skills in emergency situations, marijuana use should be avoided during child care in general.

TOLERANCE AND DEPENDENCE

Under laboratory conditions, the administration of THC several times a day for several days in humans results in tolerance to the effects of marijuana on mood, body temperature, intraocular pressure and impairment of psychomotor skills. In the real world, tolerance also develops, although many chronic users claim that they need less of the drug the more they use it. This suggests that at least some aspects of "reverse" tolerance may be due to learning. In other words, the experienced smoker has learned what effects to focus on to enhance the high. Alternatively, this effect may be due to the slow release into the blood of active metabolites stored in fatty tissue. Hence, the baseline blood levels of THC or its metabolites are greater than zero in the chronic user and thus it appears that less drug is needed to get high.

In laboratory studies, high doses of marijuana every four hours (for ten to twenty days) cause mild withdrawal symptoms when the drug is abruptly discontinued. By operational definition, this means that THC causes physical dependence. However, physical withdrawal signs are not routinely observed in patients undergoing treatment for marijuana dependence in hospitals (see Table 9.2 for symptoms of withdrawal).

Although marijuana is not as dangerous as alcohol, for example (marijuana has no major effects on the liver, heart, or gastrointestinal tract), it is addicting and produces craving, at least in some users.

TABLE 9.2: Major Symptoms of Marijuana Withdrawal in Chronic Users

- irritability
- restlessness
- insomnia
- nervousness
- decreased appetite
- weight loss
- tremor

LEGAL PENALTIES FOR MARIJUANA POSSESSION

The legal penalties for marijuana use vary greatly from state to state. Most states distinguish between possession for personal use and possession with intent to sell, which carries more severe penalties. Some states impose driver's license revocation for possession of the drug. In certain states, such as New Jersey, suspension of driving privileges is not related to driving while intoxicated or any driving act. Since the penalties associated with marijuana use vary considerably, please consult the particular laws of your state for more information.

Chapter 10

Anxiolytics:
Drugs That Calm Us Down

Anxiety is a common condition in humans who are under stress. In this chapter we will explore what happens when anxiety becomes uncontrollable and affects daily living. Antianxiety drugs (anxiolytics) have been designed to safely reduce anxiety while maintaining normal alertness. In this chapter we will explain how benzodiazepines, the prototype class of anxiolytic drugs, produce their effects when used in appropriate doses. When given to pharmacologically sensitive individuals, or in doses that are too high, or for too long a period of time, these drugs cause excessive drowsiness, dependence, and other side effects. We will review their therapeutic and nontherapeutic uses.

WHAT IS ANXIETY?

From time to time, most people experience some form of anxiety. These feelings can range from fear, to dread, to absolute terror and, depending upon the circumstances, can be perfectly normal. A major feature of clinical anxiety is that its victims do not know why they are anxious, even though their anxiety may be so severe as to be incapacitating.

Anxiety can evoke a number of autonomic nervous system responses. The responses are not under voluntary control and are part of the "fight or flight" reaction described in Chapter 1.

Charles Darwin (1809-1882), who is best known for his work on evolution, was also a very keen observer of how the perception of fear is expressed by the autonomic nervous system. Darwin's observations made over a century ago are so accurate that they are well worth repeating in this chapter.

> Fear is often preceded by astonishment . . . the senses of sight and hearing being instantly aroused. . . . The eyes and mouth are widely opened, and the eyebrows raised . . . [you stand] like a statue motionless and breathless, [crouching] instinctively to escape observation. The heart beats quickly and violently, so that it palpitates or knocks against the ribs . . . [and] the skin instantly becomes pale . . . due to the . . . contraction of the small arteries of the skin. That the skin is much affected under the sense of great fear, we see in the marvelous and inexplicable manner in which perspiration immediately exudes from it. This exudation is all the more remarkable, as the surface is then cold, and hence the term a cold sweat. . . . the hairs also on the skin stand erect; and the superficial muscles shiver . . . the heart, the breathing is hurried. The salivary glands act imperfectly; the mouth becomes dry, and is often opened and shut [and] . . . there is a strong tendency to yawn. One of the best-marked symptoms is the trembling of all the muscles of the body; and this is often first seen in the lips . . . the voice becomes husky or indistinct, or may altogether fail . . . As fear increases into an agony of terror . . . the heart beats wildly, or may fail to act and faintness ensue; there is a deathlike pallor; the breathing is labored; the wings of the nostrils are widely dilated; there is a gasping and convulsive motion of the lips, a tremor on the hollow cheek, a gulping and catching of the throat; the uncovered and protruding eyeballs are fixed on the object of terror; or they may roll restlessly from side to side. . . . The pupils are . . . enormously dilated. All the muscles of the body may become rigid, or may be thrown into convulsive movements. The hands are alternatively clenched and opened, often with a twitching movement. The arms may be protruded, as if to avert some dreadful danger, or may be thrown wildly over the head. . . . In other cases there is a sudden and uncontrollable tendency to headlong flight . . .[1]

WHAT ARE ANXIETY DISORDERS?

Anxiety disorders can include generalized anxiety disorder, panic disorder, agoraphobia (fear of venturing outside), social phobia, post-traumatic stress disorder, and obsessive-compulsive disorder. Of these, the most well studied are panic disorder, social phobia, and post-traumatic stress disorder.

Anxiety produces a variety of subjective and physical symptoms (see Table 10.1). Visceral (inside organ) effects of anxiety originate in the hypothalamic-pituitary system and may include increased plasma norepinephrine, epinephrine, and cortisol. The motor symptoms, which include shakiness, tremor, and muscular tension, arise in the extrapyramidal motor system (see Chapter 12).

Treatment of anxiety may focus on reducing physical symptoms as well as psychological triggers of anxiety. Treatment using psychoactive medication should almost always include psychotherapeutic treatment as well.

Anxiety is normal! Everyone experiences a certain amount of anxiety. Low-level anxiety is motivating and helpful. It is when anxiety is so intense that it is physically or emotionally incapacitating that it should be treated.

TABLE 10.1: Biobehavioral Symptoms of Anxiety

- hyperactivity (nervous movement)
- fearfulness
- withdrawal
- palpitations
- chest pain
- sensations of choking/smothering
- dizziness
- feelings of unreality
- paresthesia (tingling in hands or feet)
- hot/cold flashes
- sweating
- trembling/shaking
- fear of dying/going crazy or losing control
- feelings of impending doom
- dyspnea (difficulty in breathing)

WHERE DOES ANXIETY BEGIN?

Early studies of anxiety suggested that this disorder began outside the brain in the peripheral nervous system. It was believed that since the hormone adrenaline (epinephrine) stimulated the sympathetic nervous system (that part of the nervous system that responds to emergencies—the fight or flight response), anxiety was a sympathetic phenomenon. It was theorized that if you could shut off the fight or flight response, you would reduce anxiety. It was quickly learned that although many of the sympathetic nervous system responses were triggered by adrenaline, the direct infusion of this hormone did not produce subjective feelings of anxiety. This observation and other work led to the suggestion that emotions such as fear and rage were initiated in the central nervous system. We now know that all such emotions emanate from the central nervous system. Therefore, changes in emotion must be produced by altering brain chemistry. Therapists do this all the time and so do antianxiety medications.

All antianxiety medications (i.e., anxiolytics) exert their effects on the central nervous system. However, peripheral-acting drugs, such as beta blockers (e.g., propranolol) can decrease the unpleasant somatic effects associated with anxiety. Various neurotransmitter systems have been implicated in the causes of anxiety. Numerous pharmacological agents with different mechanisms of action have been employed to treat anxiety disorders. Although there is good evidence that norepinephrine and serotonin play some role in the production and treatment of anxiety disorders, the GABA system is clearly the most prominent player.

PHARMACOLOGICAL TREATMENT OF ANXIETY

Drugs used to treat anxiety are called anxiolytics, although other terms such as antianxiety drugs, minor tranquilizers (an old term), and sedatives have also been used. For the most part, these terms are interchangeable.

Drug Treatment of Anxiety

Over the centuries, various drugs have been used to treat anxiety. Alcohol is one of the oldest antianxiety drugs, and the interaction between alcohol and stress is well known. Under some circumstances and in some individuals, low doses of alcohol decrease the response to stress. However, alcohol's deleterious biomedical and psychosocial effects outweigh its overall usefulness as an anxiolytic. Phenobarbital, a sedative, was a popular antianxiety agent in the early 1900s. This barbiturate has a slow onset and long duration compared to shorter-acting barbiturates more commonly used as sleeping medications (e.g., secobarbital). Its use has declined because of a slow onset and too many side effects. However, the first true anxiolytic was chlordiazepoxide (Librium).

Development of Librium and Valium

The history and development of benzodiazepines is related more to luck than anything else. Leo Sternbach was a chemist working on developing dyes in Krakow, Poland in the 1930s. During his work, he synthesized a group of compounds known as heptodiazines. About twenty years later, Sternbach was working at Hoffman La Roche Pharmaceuticals in the United States and took a closer look at his earlier invention. As it turns out, Sternbach discovered that the drug he had synthesized twenty years earlier had sedative properties. The new drug was given an experimental name, RO 5-0690, and after considerable testing and refinement it became chlordiazepoxide (Librium). It is still popular.

In the years that followed, similar drugs were developed by Sternbach and eventually marketed. These included a type known as benzodiazepines, the best-known of which is diazepam (Valium). At one time, benzodiazepines accounted for about half of all prescriptions written in the United States! Other benzodiazepines include: oxazepam (Serax), clorazepate (Tranxene), and lorazepam (Ativan). These drugs produce mild sedation (sleepiness), anxiolytic effects, muscle relaxation, and anticonvulsant effects. Different benzodiazepines have different therapeutic purposes.

ABSORPTION, DISTRIBUTION, AND ELIMINATION

Heptodiazines and benzodiazepines are acids and are rapidly absorbed from the gastrointestinal tract. Peak blood levels can occur as quickly as thirty minutes to as long as three hours after oral administration, depending upon the specific anxiolytic. Some benzodiazepines may take up to eight hours to reach a maximum concentration in the blood, and blood levels can vary as much as twentyfold with the same dose in different people. Absorption following an oral dose is generally more rapid than by injection, since the drug tends to bind to proteins and does so more readily at an injection site than in the digestive tract. The absorption of benzodiazepines is increased by very low doses of alcohol and the combination of both drugs at high doses can be fatal.

Two Half-Lives

Benzodiazepines have a half-life from about two to ten hours, depending upon the particular drug and other factors. Much of the variation in bioavailability is because of distribution changes—the drug is easily taken up by fat tissue. The first phase of bioavailability is followed by a much slower elimination phase, with a half life of twenty-seven to forty-eight hours. Benzodiazepines have several metabolites (n-desmethyldrazepam, oxazepam) that are also psychoactive and extend the drug's effect for many more hours than the original parent compound. Therefore, the time it takes for the parent compound to reach maximum concentration (see above) may not reflect the time course for the achievement of maximum psychoactive effect. Since alcohol interferes with the metabolism of benzodiazepines and significantly increases their half life (by about 50 percent), it is dangerous to use both of these together.

HOW DO BENZODIAZEPINES WORK?

Normal GABA Functioning

Benzodiazepines interact with receptors on neurons that use the neurotransmitter gamma-aminobutyric acid (GABA) to change the functional activity of the cell. GABA acts as one of the brain's endogenous tranquilizing systems. When GABA receptors are occupied by GABA molecules, a Cl^- channel in the membrane of the cell opens, allowing ions to enter the cell and hyperpolarizing it, thus decreasing the probability of an action potential. Since this is an inhibitory action, GABA produces an IPSP (see Chapter 5). This neurochemical change, when produced in specific brain areas, is associated with relaxation and a decrease in anxiety.

In most people, behavioral states change rapidly according to environmental circumstances. The GABA system's role in such changes is governed by endogenous (made within the body) ligands, proteins synthesized in the body that bind to neurotransmitters (receptors). These ligands inhibit GABA binding, thus reversing the relaxed, anxiety-free behavioral state. There are several such endogenous ligands, one of which is called GABA modulin. GABA modulin is a recognition receptor protein located in the neuronal membrane. When activated, GABA modulin works in concert with GABA to regulate Cl^- ion flow. The GABA modulin binds to the benzodiazepine recognition protein, inhibits GABA binding, and thus closes the Cl^- ion channel, decreasing IPSPs (see Figure 10.1).

Benzodiazepines Change the GABA System

Benzodiazepine, the drug, has the opposite effect of endogenous benzodiazepine ligand; it increases the functional activity of the inhibitory amino acid neurotransmitter, GABA. By blocking the action of GABA modulin and/or other endogenous ligands, benzodiazepines increase the binding of GABA to GABA receptors and therefore increase postsynaptic IPSPs.

GABA must act as part of an anxiety-regulating network in the central nervous system. Normally, GABA binding is inhibited by one of several endogenous benzodiazepine ligands. This increases autonomic arousal and "good" anxiety. It keeps us vigilant, alert for changes in our environment, and so on. Under some conditions, which are not fully understood, this state of arousal goes out of control, causing the clinical symptoms associated with an anxiety disorder. Benzodiazepines block GABA modulin (or perhaps some other endogenous benzodiazepine ligand) and increase the postsynaptic binding of GABA. The increase in GABA receptor binding inhibits the brain's normal anxiety system.

Drugs that have effects opposite to benzodiazepines at a molecular level would be expected to increase anxiety. They do. For exam-

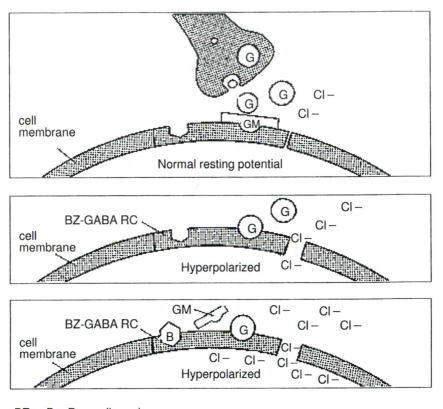

BZ or B = Benzodiazepine
GABA or G = Gamma-aminobutyric acid
BZ-GABA RC = Benzodiazepine-GABA Receptor Complex
GM = GABA Modulin

FIGURE 10.1. Benzodiazepine-GABA modulin receptor complex.

ple, caffeine blocks the benzodiazepine receptors and prevents the natural benzodiazepine ligand from having its effect. Even moderate doses of caffeine make people anxious and nervous, and this caffeine-produced anxiety cannot be treated effectively with benzodiazepines.

WHERE ARE BENZODIAZEPINE RECEPTORS?

Benzodiazepine receptors are distributed throughout the brain. The greatest concentrations are found in the frontal and occipital cortex, hypothalamus, cerebellum, midbrain, and hippocampus. Probable sites involved in benzodiazepine anxiolytic action are the septum, hippocampus, hypothalamus, and other limbic system structures.

BIOBEHAVIORAL EFFECTS OF BENZODIAZEPINES

Anxiolytics

Benzodiazepines are effective anxiolytics. The primary use of benzodiazepines is to reduce anxiety without producing profound sedation. Lorazepam (Ativan) and alprazolam (Xanax) are popular anxiolytic benzodiazepines.

Motor Disorders

For the most part, the effects of benzodiazepines are limited to the central nervous system, even though many actions of this drug are seemingly outside the central nervous system. For example, a decrease in the muscular tension associated with anxiety is one prominent beneficial effect of benzodiazepines. In high doses, these drugs are used in the treatment of motor disorders such as Parkinson's disease, multiple sclerosis, and brain injuries that produce increased muscular tone.

Seizures

Benzodiazepines also have anticonvulsant properties. For this reason they are often prescribed during alcohol detoxification when patients are seizure-prone.

Insomnia

Benzodiazepines may also be effective in treating insomnia. Flurazepam (Dalmane) is frequently used in the United States and nitrazepam (Mogadon) in Europe for this purpose. These benzodiazepines decrease the time it takes to fall asleep as well as the number of wakings during the night. Benzodiazepines decrease the amount of time spent in rapid eye movement (REM), stage III, and stage IV sleep, but this effect diminishes with use. When the drug is discontinued, there is a rebound effect (REM, insomnia) that may last for one to two weeks. Increased REM is associated with bizarre dreaming, restlessness, and frequent awakenings during the night.

Ataxia and Miscellaneous Effects

Benzodiazepines produce ataxia (lack of coordination) and drowsiness in 2 and 4 percent of the prescribed population, respectively. Occasionally, agitation, rage, aggression, depression, and sleep disorders also occur. Clinically administered for the treatment of anxiety, doses of more than 300 mg/day of Valium or 120 mg/day of Librium probably indicates another cause for anxiety, namely, abuse of the drug.

Mood and Driving

A number of studies have been performed to determine the effects of benzodiazepines on mood and psychophysical motor performance. While these studies generally suggest that benzodiazepines produce some adverse effects (e.g. confusion, fatigue, changes in simple reaction time, driving performance, etc.), the clinical significance of such findings must be interpreted cautiously for two reasons. Most such studies used only single doses of the drug, which were not administered clinically, and most studies did not use anxious subjects. Those few studies that did use anxious subjects often reported improved performance, particularly when anxiety might be expected to interfere with test performance. Few studies have examined the effects of doses well in excess of the therapeutic range. When benzodiazepines are prescribed, the effects of these drugs on performance, such as operating a motor vehicle, are not known and await further investigation.

Toxicity

Valium, one of the early benzodiazepines, has very low toxicity and does not activate liver microsomal enzymes. This means that

Valium is unlikely to alter the metabolism of other drugs and thus their toxicity. Also, in comparison to other anxiolytics, the potential for abuse, although present, is relatively low. Doses as high as 2250 mg of Librium have been reported without the deep coma and respiratory depression effects seen with other sedative-hypnotics. However, the combination of anxiolytics with alcohol can be fatal, particularly at high doses.

BENZODIAZEPINES AND THE FETUS

Like most psychoactive drugs, benzodiazepines cross the placental barrier easily and also appear in the milk of nursing mothers. Although there are little data to suggest that benzodiazepines produce birth defects, infants born of mothers using benzodiazepines at therapeutic doses show withdrawal symptoms such as tremors, irritability, and hyperactivity at birth. These are similar to opiate withdrawal. Pregnant women are thus advised not to use benzodiazepines.

ABUSE OF AND DEPENDENCE ON BENZODIAZEPINES

Benzodiazepines have been used since the early 1960s, but only recently have gained attention as having abuse potential. Early observations suggested that some heptodiazines and benzodiazepines produce withdrawal symptoms when administered in extremely high doses (100-600 mg/day, compared to therapeutic doses of 20-40 mg/day). In those case studies, withdrawal began about four to eight days after the drug was discontinued and lasted for several days. Physicians prescribing these drugs thought that since the doses used were extremely high, dependence was very unlikely at therapeutic doses. More recent studies have revealed that high (135 mg/day) and low (20 mg/day) doses were capable of producing withdrawal (see Table 10.2).

In the general population, clinical use of benzodiazepines usually does not produce significant problems. However, benzodiazepines do produce moderate dependence, especially if used over long periods or in high doses. Withdrawal from benzodiazepines is usually complicated by withdrawal from other substances.

TABLE 10.2. Benzodiazepine Withdrawal Symptoms

- anxiety
- sleep disturbances
- sensitivity to bright lights and noise
- increased auditory evoked potentials (experimental)
- weight loss
- unsteady gait
- numbness or tingling (5 days to 2 weeks after abstinence)

OTHER ANXIOLYTIC MEDICATIONS

Meprobamate (Miltown, Equanil) was another early antianxiety agent. Meprobamate is a propyl alcohol derivative with pharmacological properties similar to benzodiazepines. It reduces anxiety without the sedation associated with barbiturates, although high doses do produce widespread central nervous system depression. At first, it was thought that meprobamate was less physically addicting than barbiturates. As it turned out, it was more addicting than originally believed, especially when taken over long periods of time. However, meprobamate is a relatively safe drug and overdoses are rare even with very high doses, except when it is taken in combination with other drugs. The combination of alcohol and meprobamate, for example, can be lethal. The use of meprobamate has declined in part because of the availability of newer, longer-acting benzodiazepines.

Buspirone (BuSpar) is a novel anxiolytic that is pharmacologically distinct from benzodiazepines. Buspirone increases brain serotonin activity ($5-HT_{1a}$ agonist), has a low potential for abuse, produces little sedation or cognitive impairment, and its discontinuation is not associated with withdrawal symptoms.

GUIDELINES FOR THE USE OF ANXIOLYTIC DRUGS

1. Before prescribing, try to identify the life stressors that precipitate or aggravate anxiety that might be treated psychotherapeutically. In the case of a life event that cannot be altered by

either therapy or drugs (e.g., loss of a spouse, job), you must explain that the drug is only part of the treatment.

2. For chronic anxiety, the doses should be regulated. The patient should not use the drug "as needed" (see Table 10.3).

3. Use in combination with psychotherapy, not as a replacement for it.

4. Drug-free holidays should be encouraged. Usually a week or more is necessary to completely eliminate the drug and its active metabolites. In some cases, the use of a placebo such as a sugar tablet or a pseudoplacebo such as an antihistamine may be warranted.

5. Generally, older anxiolytics (e.g., meprobamate) are not used much anymore, because newer drugs have higher potency and require fewer doses per day for the same effect. All antianxiety drugs are useful, but different ones are used based upon patient response, physician preferences, and convenience of dosing.

TABLE 10.3. Dose Guidelines for Sedation

Benzodiazepine Derivatives

- Xanax (alprazolam) 0.25-8 mg
- Librium (chlordiazepoxide) 10-25 mg
- Tranxene (clorazepate) 7.5-15 mg
- Valium (diazepam) 5-10 mg

Chapter 11

Antidepressants:
Drugs That Lift Us Up

Almost everyone has felt some form of depression at some time in their lives. In this chapter we will discuss the difference between just feeling down and clinical depression and how antidepressants range from mild "normalizers" to powerful drugs that will help some people out of their "deep hole of clinical depression." We will see that depression has many causes, but all causes appear to be expressed through mediators of chemical deficiencies. Antidepressant drugs restore the normal chemistry of the brain, thereby making the person feel better. The therapeutic use of these drugs can bridge the depressive episode, raise the mood to allow the patient to respond to psychotherapy, and in other patients with more difficult prognoses, literally act as lifesavers.

WHAT IS DEPRESSION?

Affective disorders refer to changes in emotion or affective states. One of the most common affective disorders is depression. In this chapter, we will discuss the basic clinical symptomology of depression and therapeutic drugs used to treat it.

Everyone has experienced feelings of sadness, isolation, or helplessness. Although the word depression has been somewhat overused to describe these feelings, 3 to 4 percent of the adult population experiences true clinical depression at some time in life. It is normal to feel sad or blue from time to time, but several things distinguish these feelings from true clinical depression.

Clinical depression is more intense and more long-lasting than "the blues." In fact, true depression is often so intense and lasts for so long that it interferes with normal day-to-day functioning for weeks or months. People cannot work at their jobs or get things done around the house. Depressed persons spend a lot of time sitting around the house, perhaps watching television or eating. Extreme changes in eating behavior such as loss of appetite and associated weight loss, or compulsive eating and weight gain, are often seen in depressed individuals. In some cases, eating is decreased because it just requires too much work. Depressed persons feel as though they have no energy or strength and nothing they do will make a difference.

There are many categories of depression that are treated effectively through the use of antidepressant drugs (see Table 11.1). However, not all drugs are effective in each of the several types of depression. Why is this so? Two reasons: individual differences between subjects make them differentially responsive to treatment with these drugs, and drug treatments have different mechanisms and specificity of actions that match or do not match different underlying biochemical causes of the many forms of depression described by clinicians (see Table 11.2).

TABLE 11.1. Major Categories of Depression

- Reactive—in reaction to an external event (e.g., loss of job, loved one)
- Endogenous—no obvious precipitating cause
- Bipolar—major mood swings, manic-depression
- Psychotic—combination of schizophrenia and depression

TABLE 11.2. Biobehavioral Symptoms Associated with Depression

- sleep disturbances (e.g., insomnia, early waking, too much sleeping)
- anorexia (loss of appetite)
- agitation or retardation of psychomotor behavior
- mania (hyperactivity, paranoia, euphoria, flight of ideas)

Most theories concerning the etiology of depression are derived from the amazing effectiveness of five major classes of antidepressant drugs used to treat depression (see Table 11.3). That these drugs are so successful in treating depression and have relatively specific mechanisms of action strongly point to an underlying biochemical process in the expression of this behavioral disorder. Many antidepressant drugs alter the functional activity of brain monoamines.

TABLE 11.3. Neuropharmacology of Depression

- monoamine oxidase inhibitors
- lithium salts
- stimulants
- tricyclics
- heterocyclics

WHAT ARE MONOAMINES?

Monoamines are a group of neurochemicals characterized by having a single amine group. The most common monoamines are serotonin, norepinephrine, and dopamine (norepinephrine and dopamine are also in a separate and distinct category of neurochemicals called catecholamines).

During the 1950s, the tuberculosis sanitariums were overloaded with patients. Tuberculosis is a disease of the lungs caused by a bacterium. The early therapy consisted of confining the individual and treatment with very nonspecific drugs. In the 1950s, iproniazid was introduced. Iproniazid is an antibiotic that emptied the sanitariums except for those who were beyond recovery. The treatment with iproniazid had one interesting side effect. It caused some degree of elation on the wards. This elation was not totally unexpected (after all, the patients were cured of a terrible disease), except for its extent and persistence. It was finally realized that iproniazid was causing elation in patients who were "depressed" long before they ever had tuberculosis. The term "psychic energizer" was coined and the first antidepressants were born. By 1952, it was discovered that iproniziad's antidepressant effects were due to inhibition of the enzyme monoamine oxidase (MAO).

It was not surprising that antipsychotics and antidepressants were serendipitous discoveries. Since MAO is an enzyme involved in the oxidation of norepinephrine, dopamine, and serotonin, clinical effectiveness of this drug in treating depression suggested a biochemical etiology that involved monoamines. By blocking the breakdown of monoamines, iproniazid increased the functional activity of these neurotransmitters, suggesting (more specifically) that depression was caused by a decrease in available monoamines.

A short time later, one of the major biochemical theories of depression, the Norepinephrine Theory, was developed. Schildkraut proposed that brain norepinephrine played an important part in affective disorders and that depression was related to a decrease in endogenous norepinephrine, with mania being caused by an increase or overabundance of norepinephrine.[1] Schildkraut's theory rests primarily on clinical changes in affect following pharmacological intervention. Drugs that increase the functional activity of noradrenergic neurons are effective in alleviating clinical depression. Drugs that decrease the functional activity of these neurons lead to depression. Several categories of drugs that alter brain monoamines by increasing their functional activity are effective in treating depression.

MONOAMINE OXIDASE INHIBITORS

Monoamine oxidase is the enzyme that regulates intracellular catecholamines and thus catecholamine availability for neurotransmission. Although the postsynaptic effects of norepinephrine and dopamine are terminated primarily by their reuptake into the presynaptic membrane, the inhibition of MAO increases intracellular levels of catecholamines. MAO inhibitors (MAOIs) irreversibly and nonspecifically inactivate MAO-A and MAO-B, thereby increasing the functional activity of catecholamines. They are very successful in alleviating depression.

The most popular MAO inhibitors include phenelzine (Nardil) and iproniazid. Iproniazid is no longer used to treat depression and has been withdrawn from the market because it was found to cause liver damage. MAOIs act by forming a stable complex with monoamine oxidase, thus preventing MAO from oxidizing intracellular catecholamines. Figure 11.1 shows the similarity between several MAOIs and catecholamines. It is the structural similarity between these drugs and the naturally occurring neurotransmitters that enables the drug to bind to MAO instead of the neurotransmitter. Phenelzine and, to a greater extent, tranylcypromine (Parnate), are effective antidepressants currently available in the United States. These drugs are "third-choice" antidepressants, however, because of their many side effects, such as postural hypotension (reduced

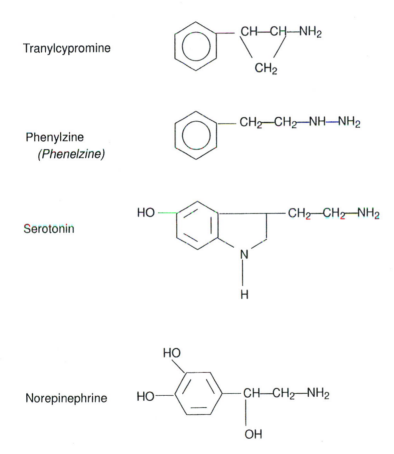

FIGURE 11.1. Structure of MAOIs and monoamines.

blood pressure upon standing), liver damage, and interaction with certain foods containing tyramine, which can lead to incidents of hypertension (high blood pressure).

LITHIUM SALTS

Lithium is sometimes prescribed as a treatment for people with symptoms of bipolar depression (episodes of mania and depression) or to treat people with unipolar depression. The exact mechanism of lithium's action is somewhat unclear. Administered as a salt, the ion could substitute for several metals such as Na^+, K^+, Mg^{++} or Ca^+ at various cellular sites. You will recall from Chapter 5 that changes in ionic flux alter neurotransmission. Lithium can increase the uptake of both tyrosine and tryptophan into synaptosomes, but its effect on catecholamine system activity is inconsistent. The nonspecificity of this drug is further indicated by its use in treating not only mania and depression but schizophrenia as well.

STIMULANTS

Early drug treatment for depression relied on stimulants that increased the functional activity of catecholamines. Although such stimulants as cocaine and amphetamine or methylphenidate are useful in short-term treatment (i.e., a few days) of exogenous depression and to improve mood in nondepressed individuals, they do not provide satisfactory improvement in clinical depression that may last for weeks, months, or longer. Moreover, such drugs have a high potential for abuse and addiction.

TRICYCLIC ANTIDEPRESSANTS

Drugs in this class increase the functional activity of norepinephrine, dopamine, and serotonin by inhibiting the reuptake of these monoamines, thereby increasing their availability and activity in the synapse. Since these drugs all have a three-ring molecular structure, they are called tricyclic antidepressants. Imipramine (Tofranil) has been found to have an equal effect on the reuptake of serotonin and norepinephrine, whereas desipramine (Norpramin) is more specific to norepinephrine, and amitriptyline (Elavil) is more specific to serotonin. Although all of these are effective antidepressants, one may be more effective than the other in individual cases, based upon the clinical response of each depressive. It is also logical that lethargy and symptoms of retarded psychomotor behavior may be better treated with a tricyclic that primarily affects norepinephrine. A new class of four-ring compounds, tetracyclics, has recently been introduced for the treatment of depression. An example of a tetracyclic antidepressant is maprotiline (Ludiomil).

SELECTIVE SEROTONIN REUPTAKE INHIBITORS

From the beginning of the Golden Age of Pharmacology, serotonin was believed to be an important neurochemical in depression. In recent years, scientists have developed selective serotonin reuptake inhibitors (SSRIs). Rather than increasing the functional activity of brain serotonin by inhibiting MAO, these drugs selectively inhibit serotonin reuptake, unlike the nonselective mechanism by which tricyclics alter norepinephrine, dopamine, and serotonin. These drugs are now the mainstay of current antidepressant therapy. The most famous of these compounds is fluoxetine (Prozac). Others that have gained popularity include fluvoxamine (Luvox), sertraline (Zoloft), and paroxetine (Paxil). All are slightly different in their clinical indications and side effects. In general, their side effects are not as uncomfortable as those of other antidepressants. Normal serotonergic neurotransmission is illustrated in Figure 11.2.

OTHER MEDICATIONS

Drugs with mixed serotonin effects, such as trazodone (Desyrel) and nefazodone (Serzone) are still being evaluated for their exact place in the treatment of depression and other disorders. A mixed norepinephrine/dopamine uptake inhibitor, bupropion (Wellbutrin),

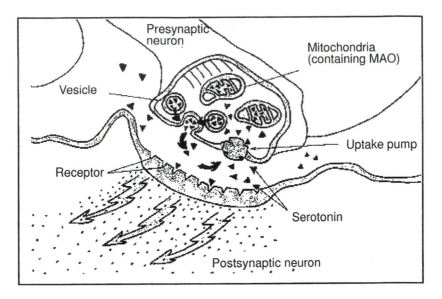

FIGURE 11.2. Normal serotonergic neurotransmission. Modified from Prozac: Comprehensive Monograph, Eli Lilly and Co. Used with permission.

is a popular antidepressant that is also being used in the treatment of alcohol dependence and for smoking cessation (Zyban). A final combined mechanism of action (serotonin/norepinephrine uptake inhibitor) is being tried in the form of venlafaxine (Effexor). This drug might be useful in treating patients who need a boost in synaptic norepinephrine and serotonin. See Table 11.4 for a list of antidepressants.

Several antidepressants, such as zimeldine (an SSRI) and nomifensine have been taken off the U.S. market because of dangerous side effects (liver toxicity).

Antidepressants are nonaddicting. They work on different brain areas than the addicting drugs such as alcohol, nicotine, cocaine, and heroin. They *can* be abused, but abuse is rare, and withdrawal is minimal. Tolerance can occur in some people, but impaired control is also very rare.

TABLE 11.4. Frequently Prescribed Antidepressants

Generic Name	Trade Name	Initial Dose (mg)*	Elimination Half-Life (hr.)
Tricyclics			
Imipramine	Tofranil	50-75	6-34
Amitriptyline	Elavil	50-75	9-46
Trimipramine	Surmontil	50-75	7-40
Doxepin	Sinequan	50-75	8-36
Desipramine	Norpramin	50-75	11-46
Nortriptyline	Pamelor	25-50	16-88
Protriptyline	Vivactil	10-20	54-198
Amoxapine	Asendin	50-150	8-30
SSRIs			
Fluoxetine	Prozac	10-20	24-120
Fluvoxamine	Luvox	50	15-26
Paroxetine	Paxil	20	24-31
Sertraline	Zoloft	50	27
MAOIs			
Phenelzine	Nardil	15	1.5-4
Tranylcypromine	Parnate	20	1.5-3
Mixed Serotonin Effects			
Trazodone	Desyrel	50-150	6-11
Nefazodone	Serzone	200	2-4
Mixed reuptake inhibitors			
Bupropion (Norepinephrine, dopamine)	Wellbutrin	200	10-21
Venlafaxine (Serotonin, norepinephrine)	Effexor	75	5

* Doses used in clinical practice may be higher or lower than indicated, depending on patient's needs.

Chapter 12

Antipsychotics: Drugs That Make Us Sane

Major psychoses such as manic depression (bipolar illness) or schizophrenia are brain diseases that are not the fault of the victim. While many factors are involved in these psychopathologies, the primary causes appear to be disruptions of brain chemistry in parts of the brain dealing with sensory perception and mood. Before the advent of the Golden Age of Pharmacology of the 1950s, the best we could do for psychotic patients was to give them high doses of alcohol, bromides, or morphine. In this chapter, we will discuss current drug therapies that involve more sophisticated, more specific, and less toxic compounds to normalize mood and reduce delusions and hallucinations. Nevertheless, psychoses are still not managed as effectively as we would like, and this area remains a frontier for the sciences of neurobiology and neuropharmacology. Let's take a closer look at the psychopharmacology of psychosis.

WHAT IS PSYCHOSIS?

Of all the behaviors in the human repertoire, the various forms of psychosis such as schizophrenia, schizoaffective disorder, affective disorders with psychosis, etc., are probably the most bizarre, the most interesting, and the most baffling. Psychoses are complex, sometimes culturally confounded disorders whose diagnoses are based upon a constellation of symptoms, rather than a single behavior. If you have not personally worked with schizophrenics (for example), it may be difficult to fully appreciate the treatment advances provided by psychotherapeutic medications.

Schizophrenia is prototypical and the most complex of all psychoses. Broadly defined, schizophrenia may be acute or chronic. Acute schizophrenia has a sudden onset with full-blown symptoms but a good prognosis. Chronic schizophrenia has a gradual onset, the symptoms become progressively worse, and the prognosis is poor. Generally, schizophrenics have disturbances concerning reality testing and concept formation with the following symptoms and categories.

SYMPTOMS OF SCHIZOPHRENIA

Thinking and Speech Disturbances

Schizophrenics have paralogical thinking, distortions of memory, perplexity, and confusion, often with feelings of unusual power. They may speak in rhymes using made-up words (neologisms) or use monotonous repetitive words or sentences. Some schizophrenics may be mute, whereas others may talk constantly. Schizophrenics have delusions of influence, grandeur, persecution, or reference.

Catatonic Motor Behavior

Some schizophrenics have motor disturbances. These patients may remain in rigid, unusual positions for extended periods of time. Often, in their delusion, they may believe that the balance of democracy and the free world as we know it is dependent upon their posture.

Schizophrenic Hallucinations

Auditory as well as other hallucinations may be present. Usually patients hear voices of real or imaginary people who talk to, threaten, accuse, curse, or criticize them. "Visions" may be of angels and devils. Hallucinations of smell, taste, and touch often occur. Some patients may experience peculiar sensations in their genitals caused by some "other."

Disturbances of Affect and Emotion

Some forms of schizophrenia include flatness of emotion or inappropriate emotion. Acute schizophrenics frequently manifest anxieties and fears resulting in excitement and panic, or they may show depression, apathy, or lethargy. Emotional behaviors are often combined with confused thinking, perplexity, fearful dream states, and dissociative phenomena (e.g., disturbances in identity, memory, or consciousness).

Disturbances of Social Behavior

These disturbances are characterized by social deterioration and sometimes complete regression from social contact. In some cases, even attention to bodily functions deteriorates (e.g., eating, urinating, defecating, personal appearance, and cleanliness). Unpredictable giggling, silly behavioral mannerisms, aggression, and loss of interest in intellectual and social pursuits may also be symptoms of schizophrenia.

Some of these symptoms may sound similar to descriptions of people under the influence of some illicit drugs or in the end stages of addiction. There are some remarkable similarities in the neuropharmacology of intoxication and psychotic behavior, but do not jump to the conclusion that intoxication is the cause of psychosis! Let's take a closer look at what the treatment of schizophrenia has taught us about the neurochemical cause of this disease.

EARLY TREATMENTS FOR SCHIZOPHRENIA

Schizophrenia is not a new disease, and early treatments were crude, to say the least. Cold-water dunking, bleeding patients with leeches, or burning them at the stake were common. Less than a hundred years ago, straitjackets and other restraints were considered acceptable treatments. About fifty years ago, insulin-induced coma, electroconvulsive shock, and psychosurgery were also used routinely to treat this disease. All that changed with the advent of two drugs that began the Golden Age of Pharmacology.

GOLDEN AGE OF PHARMACOLOGY

Coincidentally, in the 1950s, two drugs were introduced in the treatment of schizophrenia. The first was reserpine (Serpasil), which destroys the vesicles that store monoaminergic neurotransmitters. In short, the first antipsychotic medication was a monoaminergic antagonist. It calmed the schizophrenic, restoring behavior to a normal degree without causing significant sedation. Reserpine's use was short-lived, however, because a second, more effective drug, chlorpromazine, was introduced at about the same time.

Chlorpromazine (Thorazine) was developed in France as part of a study of hibernation. Chlorpromazine does indeed lower body temperature and exerts a quieting effect on the subject. However, in searching for a drug that would reduce preoperative anxiety, scientists found that chlorpromazine made normal patients indifferent about the upcoming operation. Eventually, the drug was tested in schizophrenics and produced similar results (it causes a selective reduction in abnormal behavior with only mild sedation). At doses that would not alter the behavior of a normal individual, chlorpromazine quiets the psychotic episodes of schizophrenics. Furthermore, it has fewer side effects than reserpine and a very high therapeutic index. Chlorpromazine soon replaced reserpine as the drug of choice in the treatment of schizophrenia. Soon thereafter, it was discovered that chlorpromazine has a major effect on dopamine in the brain (Figure 12.1).

Interestingly, psychiatric hospital records between 1900 and 1955 reveal that the number of beds occupied by psychiatric patients had increased steadily. Immediately following the introduction of reserpine and chlorpromazine, the number of hospital beds occupied by psychiatric patients declined dramatically. These data suggested quite convincingly that schizophrenia is a biological disorder best treated by a neuropharmacological approach.

Phenothiazine Antipsychotics

Chlorpromazine is the prototype for a number of phenothiazine antipsychotic drugs (see Table 12.1). Many of these are still in use today.

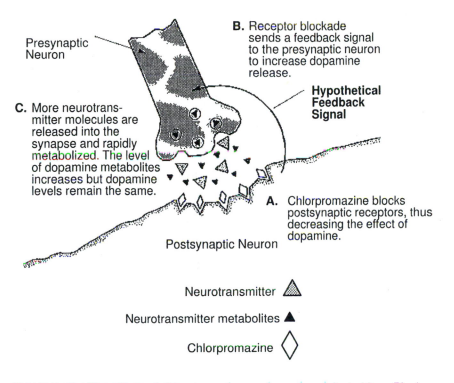

B. Receptor blockade sends a feedback signal to the presynaptic neuron to increase dopamine release.

Presynaptic Neuron

Hypothetical Feedback Signal

C. More neurotransmitter molecules are released into the synapse and rapidly metabolized. The level of dopamine metabolites increases but dopamine levels remain the same.

A. Chlorpromazine blocks postsynaptic receptors, thus decreasing the effect of dopamine.

Postsynaptic Neuron

Neurotransmitter △

Neurotransmitter metabolites ▲

Chlorpromazine ◇

FIGURE 12.1.The effects of chlorpromazine on dopamine. Adapted from Pinel, 1989.[1]

Other Antipsychotics

Clozapine and loxapine are dibenzodiazepines. Like phenothiazines, they block dopamine receptors but somewhat weakly. Interestingly, clozapine also blocks serotonin, norepinephrine, histamine, and acetylcholine receptors, which may explain why it is often effective in treating patients who are resistant to typical dopamine antagonist antipsychotics. Although useful because it has relatively few side effects compared to other antipsychotic medications, clozapine does increase risk for seizures, and sedation, and decreases white blood cell count (agranulocytosis).

TABLE 12.1. Major Categories and Commonly Prescribed Antipsychotics

Drug	Trade Name[1]	Route	Dosage Range (mg)[2]	Sedation[4]	Extra Effects Autonomic[3]	Extra Effects Pyramidal
Phenothiazines						
Chlorpromazine	Thorazine	Oral, IM	60-2000	***	***	**
Fluphenazine	Prolixin	Oral, IM	2-40	*	*	***
Trifluoperazine	Stelazine	Oral, IM	2-80	**	*	***
Perphenazine	Trilafon	Oral, IM	8-64	**	*	***
Thioridazine	Mellaril	Oral	50-800	***	***	**
Butyrophenones						
Haloperidol	Haldol	Oral, IM	1-100	*	*	***
Thioxanthenes						
Thiothixene	Navane	Oral, IM	5-60	*	**	***
Dihydroindolones						
Molindone	Moban	Oral	15-225	*	*	**
Dibenzoxazepines						
Loxapine	Loxitane	Oral, IM	20-250	**	**	***
Clozapine	Clozaril	Oral	75-900	****	***	*
Benzisoxazole						
Risperidone	Risperdal	Oral	2-16	*	**	**

1. Original trade name. Others are available, plus generic forms.
2. Doses used in clinical practice may be higher or lower than indicated based on patient needs.
3. Most common autonomic side effect is hypotension.
4. Number of asterisks indicates severity of side effects.

Antipsychotic medications decrease agitation, paranoia, and delusions without producing euphoria. However, many patients find the side effects of antipsychotics unpleasant and "poison."

NEUROTRANSMITTERS AND SCHIZOPHRENIA

As with other psychoactive drugs, antipsychotics exert their effect on behavior by altering the functional activity of brain neurochemicals. The effectiveness of early antipsychotic medications quickly and clearly pointed to the role of brain dopamine in this mental illness. The symptoms of schizophrenia result from a biological imbalance within the brain's dopamine system. Although we still do not know precisely what aspect of the dopaminergic system is overactive, we now have some exciting insights (see Figure 12.2).

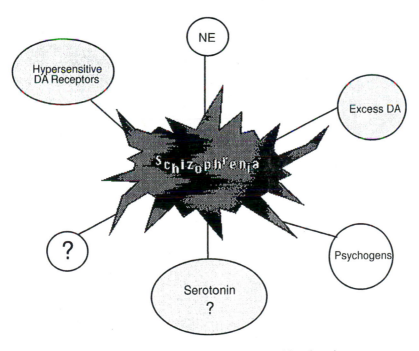

FIGURE 12.2. Multifactor model of schizophrenia.

Schizophrenia and Excess Brain Dopamine

The most convincing evidence for the dopamine theory of schizophrenia is the consistent observation that drugs that antagonize the dopamine system are effective in reducing schizophrenic behavior. Similarly, chronic high doses of drugs such as amphetamine or cocaine that activate the dopaminergic system produce schizophrenic-like behavior in the otherwise normal individual. If schizophrenic-like behavior is a disorder reflecting an overactive dopamine system, what is the physiological basis for this overactivity? Although there are many interesting approaches to answer this question, we will discuss only a few.

Too Much Dopamine?

The first possibility is that the brain of the schizophrenic has too much dopamine. This is certainly the simplest explanation. In spite of numerous attempts to measure this, however, there remains no convincing evidence that even a subpopulation of schizophrenics have too much dopamine in their brains.

Excess Dopamine Receptors?

The next possibility is that there are too many dopamine receptors in the brain of the schizophrenic. Many of the earlier studies of this hypothesis were confounded by the use of antipsychotic medications, since these drugs will increase the number of dopamine receptors. However, dopamine receptor binding studies using postmortem brain tissue from schizophrenics versus a matched set of controls show that schizophrenics do, in fact, have more dopamine receptor sites than nonschizophrenics. The inference is that a little dopamine goes a lot further in the schizophrenic.

Role of Monoamine Oxidase

Other approaches to the overactive dopamine system are also producing exciting findings. It appears that schizophrenics have much lower levels of activity of monoamine oxidase, an enzyme that metabolizes dopamine. Therefore, in patients with low enzyme levels, dopamine would be present for longer periods of time in the brains of the schizophrenic. Blood platelets also contain the enzyme monoamine oxidase. Since schizophrenics have low platelet MAO, this may be a useful biological marker for this disease.

Endogenous Psychogens (Naturally Present Schizophrenia-Producing Chemicals)

Some scientists have theorized that the brains of schizophrenics are producing an unusual dopamine agonist, phenylethylamine. Phenylethylamine is a dopaminergic agonist, an amphetamine-like stimulant normally found in low concentrations in brain tissue. Some investigators have observed unusually high concentrations of phenylethylamine in the brains of schizophrenics. Interest in endogenous psychogens, allergens, and similar chemicals has waned over the years because research in this area has not been very productive.

Abnormal Norepinephrine Metabolism May Alter Brain Dopamine

Schizophrenia may also be a disease caused by the destruction of brain norepinephrine-containing neurons resulting in an abnormal metabolism of dopamine in schizophrenics. Why? Because normally dopamine is metabolized to norepinephrine by the enzyme dopamine-beta-hydroxylase (DBH). There is some evidence that schizophrenics have lowered DBH activity, which leads to an increased accumulation of dopamine.

Role for Serotonin

There have also been studies suggesting that schizophrenia is related to the indolamine serotonin (5HT). This notion was based on the observed fluctuations in urinary levels of serotonin's major acid metabolite, 5-HIAA. When schizophrenic symptoms were at their worst, the excretion of these compounds also increased. When patients showed remission from schizophrenia, the urinary levels decreased. Since many hallucinogenic drugs have a chemical structure similar to serotonin and one of the hallmarks of schizophrenia is hallucinations, this theory is quite interesting and appealing. Support for an indolamine theory of schizophrenia comes from clinical studies showing that when dietary amino acids such as tryptophan are given to patients previously treated with MAOIs, it exacerbates schizophrenic symptoms. Yet in normal individuals, tryptophan loading usually has a sedativelike effect.

WHERE IN THE BRAIN DO ANTIPSYCHOTIC MEDICATIONS WORK?

To date, the dopamine hypothesis of schizophrenia is the best-accepted explanation of this disease, and is based on the fact that drugs that block dopamine receptors effectively treat the symptoms of this disease in the majority of patients. Antipsychotic effectiveness is directly related to the drug's ability to block a specific subtype of dopamine receptor, called the D_2 receptor. Most antipsychotic drugs currently on the market have a very high affinity for this receptor. The greater the drug's ability to bind to D_2 receptors, the more clinically effective it seems to be. These observations offer strong support for the role of dopamine in psychosis. However, it remains to be determined why such medications require several days or longer before clinical improvement occurs, particularly when these drugs block most D_2 receptors within hours of their administration. Why is this? Let's examine the parts of this puzzle and see if there is a logical solution.

First, antipsychotic medications not only block dopamine receptors, they also increase plasma homovanillic acid (HVA), a metabolite of dopamine. This increase in levels of HVA is only seen during the first few days of antipsychotic treatment; then, plasma levels decline. However, it is not until the plasma levels of HVA decrease that clinical improvement is observed. There is some evidence that patients with higher levels of HVA prior to treatment respond better to antipsychotic medication than subjects with low pretreatment HVA levels.

Second, when animals are given dopamine receptor blockers, there is an initial increase in the release of midbrain dopamine, measured electrophysiologically as an increase in cell firing rates.

This is followed by a long-term decrease in cell firing called "depolarization inactivation."[2] These results are consistent with the interpretation of changes in human plasma HVA. See Figure 12.2.

WHAT IT ALL MEANS

The brain is a remarkable organ that compensates for many changes, including the effects of antipsychotics. First, antipsychotics decrease postsynaptic dopamine activity resulting in the release of additional presynaptic dopamine (hence, HVA levels increase). Eventually, there is a decrease in dopamine activity days or weeks later and clinical improvement is observed.

Since antipsychotics block pre- and postsynaptic receptors, they probably alter a compensatory mechanism within the dopamine system. For example, the blockade of presynaptic receptors, which would regulate release, may lead to unrestricted release of dopamine, largely through an increase in the activity of tyrosine hydroxylase, an enzyme that regulates the manufacture of dopamine. This would offset the postsynaptic (therapeutic) action of the drug until the system readjusted to the presynaptic action. Eventually the medication will exert clinical as well as pharmacological effects.

Alternatively, postsynaptic blockade may result in the disinhibition of whatever other brain systems were innervated by dopamine. This would then result in an excitatory feedback loop to dopamine neurons, increasing their release and delaying for days or weeks the antipsychotic benefit of postsynaptic dopamine receptor blockade.

Although more than one neurochemical system is almost certainly involved in schizophrenia, let's examine the neuroanatomy of the brain dopamine system to see where antipsychotic medications exert their effects of the symptoms of schizophrenia.

BRAIN DOPAMINE PATHWAYS

There are at least four major dopamine pathways (Table 12.2) in the brain where antipsychotics work. The anatomy and physiology of each is discussed in detail below.

TABLE 12.2. Major Dopamine Pathways

- mesolimbic tract
- nigrostriatal tract
- mesocortical tract
- hypothalamic-pituitary (tuberoinfundibular) tract

- *Mesolimbic system:* Dopamine neurons located in the midbrain project axons to the limbic system where dopamine is released to regulate emotional behavior. Dopamine receptor supersensitivity in this area of the brain may mediate the psychomotor agitation, sensitivity to sensory stimuli, delusions, and hallucinations that often define schizophrenia. Stimulation or surgical ablation of some limbic system structures have been reported to produce behavioral and perceptual changes similar to those observed in schizophrenics.

  Finally, the mesolimbic system has a high concentration of dopamine receptors and high postmortem dopamine binding. Electroencephalograph, brain imaging, and cerebral blood flow studies reveal differences between schizophrenics and normal subjects. Taken together, there is good scientific evidence that the mesolimbic dopamine system is the key site of action for antipsychotic medications.

- *Nigrostriatal system:* Dopamine neurons from the substantia nigra region of the midbrain project to the caudate-putamen of the basal ganglia or neostriatum. The terminals of these dopamine neurons project to other neostriatal neurons that are probably cholinergic. This pathway involves muscle control and movement. Damage to the nigrostriatal pathway or cell bodies within the striatum results in Parkinson's disease. Disturbances in the motor functions are a side effect of dopamine receptor blockade, similar to Parkinsonism. The basal ganglia mediate slow voluntary movements. The extrapyramidal dopamine system regulates motor commands sent down from the cortex. Chronic blockade of dopamine receptors in this area results in extrapyramidal side effects (see below).

- *Mesocortical system:* Dopamine pathways from the midbrain to the cortex mediate the sedative effects of antipsychotic medications.
- *Hypothalamic-pituitary system:* The hypothalamus is in direct neural and circulatory contact with the pituitary gland and regulates the release of hormones. The hypothalamus, another limbic system structure, is also involved in emotion, eating, drinking, sex, and pleasure. Many pathways from the hypothalamus use dopamine to communicate information and regulate physiology and behavior.

SIDE EFFECTS

Dopamine blockade, the primary action produced by antipsychotics, interrupts many of these functions, producing side effects. For example, dopamine is a prolactin-inhibiting factor, which inhibits the release of the hormone prolactin. Since prolactin is normally involved in breast development and lactation (milk let-down), one side effect of antipsychotic medications is that they often cause breast enlargement in males (gynecomastia) and lactation in women. Other side effects of some antipsychotics include impaired ejaculation in men, loss of orgasm, abnormal menstrual cycles, or infertility in women.

Pharmacological treatment is always a cost-benefit equation. Although these drugs are effective in reducing psychotic behavior in most cases, they have associated risks. These risks involve side effects caused by the drug's unwanted actions on dopamine pathways outside the mesolimbic system. In addition to the endocrine side effects discussed above, the most profound consequence of long-term dopamine receptor blockade is on motor systems of the brain that are controlled in part by the extrapyramidal system. Many antipsychotic medications, such as Haldol, also bind to and block muscarinic or cholinergic receptors (anticholinergic effects). Generally, the more anticholinergic effects, the fewer extrapyramidal effects. See Table 12.3 for anticholinergic side effects.

Schizophrenia and Parkinson's Disease

We learned earlier that through the nigrostriatal dopamine system there was a relationship between antipsychotic drug use and Parkin-

TABLE 12.3. Anticholinergic Side Effects

- dry mouth
- blurred vision
- glaucoma
- mydriasis (pupil dilation)
- constipation
- urinary retention
- tachycardia

son's disease. Since antipsychotics decrease the functional activity of brain dopamine and Parkinsonism is a disease characterized, generally, by a hypoactive dopamine system, it should not be surprising that antipsychotic medications produce Parkinson-like behaviors including tremor and rigidity. Antipsychotic medications cause extrapyramidal side effects as well as a neuroleptic malignant syndrome (see below).

Extrapyramidal Side Effects

The pyramidal motor system is responsible for motor movements and consists of long monosynaptic pathways from the cortex, where movement is initiated, to the spinal cord, where the pathways synapse with the motor neurons that ultimately innervate muscles. The extrapyramidal system is responsible for smoothing out motor movements and producing postural changes to accommodate movements. The extrapyramidal system consists of the cortex and several subcortical structures including the basal ganglia (caudate nucleus and putamen) and the globus pallidus. Several thalamic nuclei as well as brainstem reticular formation neurons also make up the extrapyramidal system. However, when the pyramidal system is damaged, motor movement can still be initiated, suggesting that the extrapyramidal system has a much more significant role in movement. Long-term use of antipsychotics produce four types of motor disorders involving the extrapyramidal system (see Table 12.4).

TABLE 12.4. Drug-Induced Extrapyramidal System Disorders

- pseudoparkinsonism
- tardive dyskinesia
- akathisias
- acute dystonic reactions

- *Pseudoparkinsonism:* Symptoms include drooling, shuffling, pill-rolling movements of the fingers, tremor, and rigidity. The overall symptomatology may be confused with depression and the side effects are severe enough to be a common cause of noncompliance. Extreme rigidity can be associated with fever and death (see Neuroleptic Malignant Syndrome, below). Symptoms develop five to thirty days after treatment and can be nearly identical to true Parkinson's disease.
- *Tardive dyskinesia:* Symptoms include lip smacking, chewing, blowing, blepharospasm (squinting), bon-bon sign (twisting movement of tongue in cheek), and choreoatheoid (dancelike) movements of hands, fingers, toes, and body. Tardive dyskinesia is prevalent in 15 to 20 percent of patients, with more among institutionalized patients. The symptoms may subside with discontinuation of treatment or be suppressed by increasing the dose of the neuroleptic. Anticholinergics and dopamine agonists make symptoms worse.
- *Akathisias:* This is the most common extrapyramidal side effect of antipsychotic treatment. The patient feels restless, and is unable to sit comfortably without continuous motor activity. Symptoms are often mistaken for agitation. It is most common in women and the symptoms develop within three months after the initiation of treatment, but often much earlier.
- *Acute dystonic reactions:* These include facial grimacing or muscle spasms of the tongue, face, neck, and back. Symptoms are seen one to two weeks after treatment but may occur sooner.

Anticholinergic drugs are useful in treating the tremor and rigidity of pseudoparkinsonism but aggravate tardive dyskinesias.

Neuroleptic Malignant Syndrome

The neuroleptic malignant syndrome includes symptoms of severe rigidity, fever, autonomic nervous system dysregulation, and elevated heart enzymes (e.g., creatine phosphokinase). The syndrome is twice as common among men as women. A full clinical picture develops rapidly once the syndrome starts. The neuroleptic malignant syndrome is potentially lethal and requires immediate medical treatment (e.g., discontinue treatment and administer dopamine agonists such as bromocriptine).

Half-Life

Most antipsychotic drugs have fairly long elimination half-lives, most in the range of twenty to forty hours; thus, they can be given in once-a-day doses. Metabolites of these drugs can be detected in the urine for several months after drug discontinuation.

Again, these drugs can be abused, but they are not addicting. They do not produce a high, let alone impaired control, and so are not considered to be addicting. Remember, tolerance and withdrawal have nothing to do with dependence or addiction.

Chapter 13

Addiction Is Not What You Think

The field of addiction has no shortage of theories about the etiology of drug use or addiction. There are a number of catch-all terms such as the "biopsychosocioeconomic" basis for drug abuse. In the search to explain complex phenomena, theorists have tended to generalize. For example, many people think that anything that makes you feel good can be addicting (chocolate, caffeine, sex, nicotine, television). In fact, the term "addiction" has lost its scientific meaning over the years. Clinicians and scientists now use more precise, less emotion-laden terminology to describe the condition of an "inability to stop using a drug." We're not talking about "not wanting to stop"; rather, we're describing a disease state in which the patient <u>cannot</u> stop using a drug, even when the desire to stop is strong. Throughout this book, we have focused on the physiological substrates of behavior. We believe strongly, as do many other scientists, that addiction is a disease state caused by a brain chemistry imbalance in a part of the brain known as the "pleasure pathway." Of course, not all drug users are dependent; some simply use too much too often. In this final chapter, we will review some historical definitions and features of addiction and discuss how neurochemical dysfunction fits with current clinical definitions of addiction.

DEFINITIONS

Major misunderstandings exist among professionals and the general public about the definitions of terms such as addiction, chemical dependency, substance abuse, physiological dependence, and drug misuse. Actually, according to the *Diagnostic and Statistical Manual of Mental Disorders*, fourth edition (DSM-IV),[1] there are only two major classifications of drug problems:

1. Drug abuse (misuse)—in which the drug is used by choice, but in illegal or unsafe situations, or at inappropriate times or places, or in cases where the drug use is harmful to oneself or others, and
2. Drug dependence—a condition now synonymous with "drug addiction," in which there are episodes of loss of control over use of the drug, and apparent inability to modify drug use in spite of adverse consequences. An extreme example of drug dependence is a man who drinks a quart of alcohol daily, cannot hold a job, has lost his family because of constant drunkenness, and is vomiting blood several times a day. When a doctor tells the man that the alcohol is causing bleeding in his esophagus, the man still cannot stop drinking. (Alcoholism is a drug dependence.) Other examples of "impaired control" are less obvious, more difficult to diagnose, and less severe forms of the disease.

Notice that the primary characteristic of dependence (addiction) is impaired control over use of the drug. Regardless of the stories and predicaments involving drug use reported by addicted people, the one recurring theme is that once they start using the drug, they can't consistently stop. If one frequently breaks promises to oneself or others about the use of a drug, then one is likely addicted to the substance.

Researchers at the National Institute on Alcohol Abuse and Alcoholism (NIAAA) recently used data from the 1992 National Longitudinal Alcohol Epidemiologic Survey and found a significant co-occurrence of alcohol and drug use disorders in the general population. The prevalence of lifetime alcohol use disorders was 18.2 percent, with 4.9 percent and 13.3 percent of the respondents classified as alcohol abusers and alcohol dependent, respectively. For all drugs combined (not including alcohol), slightly fewer respondents were classified with dependence (2.9 percent) than with abuse (3.1 percent). This provides a general picture of the incidences of abuse versus dependence in the general population.

Many people are confused by the above new classifications, because they still remember the old definition of addiction formulated by the World Health Organization (WHO) in 1950. This definition is no longer valid. The old definition stated that an addicting drug had three qualities: (1) psychological dependence (roughly, habituation or "craving"), (2) tolerance (adaptation to the drug so that more and more is needed to produce the original effect), and (3) physical dependence. (Adaptation of the body to the drug so that one can only function normally when the drug is present. When the person stops using, the body's adaptation is observed through physical withdrawal symptoms.) While this definition properly describes dependence on central nervous system drugs such as heroin and alcohol, it falls short of describing dependence on cocaine, a central nervous system stimulant that has no significant physical withdrawal. (Up to 95 percent of withdrawal is emotional, rather than physical.) Even today, some argue that cocaine is not addicting because of this lack of physical withdrawal—a dangerous assumption. (However, it is also possible to interpret withdrawal from cocaine as having a physiological basis, since emotions and behavior are the result of changes in neurochemical function in the brain.)

Today, with our new definition of addiction, impaired control over drug use properly defines all drugs that are addicting. The new term "dependence" (addiction) still has both psychological and physical characteristics, but they are different from the old WHO definition—"impaired control" is an obsessive preoccupation with the use of the drug (psychological), and the primary cause of impaired control is a neurochemical (physical) dysfunction in the brain. Impaired control is what is seen, but neurochemistry is what is happening. (Note: it is now easy to understand that the term "substance abuse treatment center" is an inaccurate description of hospitals where chemical dependency is treated. Also, the terms "physical addiction" and "psychological addiction" really have no accurate meaning, according to DSM-IV guidelines. Finally, tolerance and physical withdrawal are side effects usually associated with moderate to heavy drug consumption, not rigid criteria for diagnosing chemical dependency—since drug abusers can also demonstrate these adaptive consequences of drug use.)

NEUROCHEMICAL DYSFUNCTION AS A CAUSE OF ADDICTIONS

Neuroscientists who study the brain now believe that the site of action of all addicting drugs probably lies within the mesolimbic system of the brain, where our instinctual drives and ability to experience emotions and pleasure reside (see Figure 13.1). Within the mesolimbic system is the medial forebrain bundle (MFB), popularly known as the pleasure pathway. The MFB runs from the center of the brain (in an area known as the ventral tegmental area, VTA), through the area above the pituitary gland (known as the lateral hypothalamus, LH), through a major "relay station" known as the nucleus accumbens (ACC), and up to the front part of the brain, known as the frontal cortex (FC). These areas, as well as several other nerve pathways that feed into them, have been well documented in animals (see Figure 13.1).

Regardless of the complexity of the pleasure pathway as it unfolds in continuing studies in neuroscience laboratories, scientists now believe that all drugs and social experiences that produce pleasure act on this pathway. In particular, drugs such as heroin, alcohol, and nicotine are known to act at least partially on the VTA to produce euphoria. Drugs acting on the ACC include cocaine, heroin (secondary site), nicotine, phencyclidine (PCP, "angel dust"), and tetrahydrocannabinol. These probable sites of drug action have been found in animal studies within the past decade, and are continually being refined and updated with new research.

All of these drugs produce euphoria and craving. But many clinicians believe that euphoria and craving alone are insufficient to produce the impaired control over drug use that characterizes drug dependence (addiction). An interesting hypothesis proposed by some scientists[2] suggests that "like-want" pathways in the MFB are intimately involved in the tolerance to euphoria and the enhanced craving that occurs in a chronic drug user. While this hypothesis provides an interesting explanation of the causes of drug abuse, it has been speculated that the MFB will soon be found to have another func-

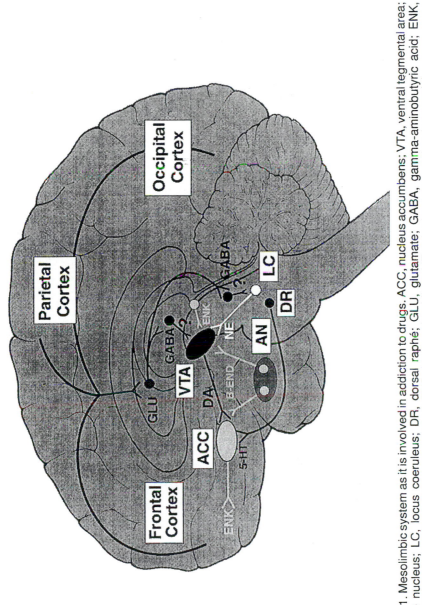

FIGURE 13.1. Mesolimbic system as it is involved in addiction to drugs. ACC, nucleus accumbens; VTA, ventral tegmental area; AN, arcuate nucleus; LC, locus coeruleus; DR, dorsal raphé; GLU, glutamate; GABA, gamma-aminobutyric acid; ENK, enkephalin; NE, norepinephrine; DA, dopamine; β-END, beta endorphin; 5-HT, 5-hydroxytryptamine (serotonin).

tional pathway, termed the "need" pathway. This need pathway could be active, because of neurochemical dysfunction, in the drug addict who cannot stop using the drug in spite of adverse consequences. The instinctual need for the drug explains the impaired control, since the person perceives the drug as intimately connected with existence, much like breathing, thirst, hunger, and the drive for sex. Thus, when they report they "can't stop" drinking or drugging, they really can't stop without professional help. Many alcoholics and other chemically-dependent people truly want to stop, but cannot do so on their own. In general, alcohol or other drug abusers will stop when they feel that life events or consequences of drinking or using are too overwhelming, and that they would be better off as social users or abstainers. There are numerous anecdotal stories of people who have stopped of their own volition, so by definition, they are not drug-dependent. (If people use alcohol or other psychoactive drugs to excess and never desire or try to stop, then by default they are usually labeled drug-dependent—but they will also probably never receive treatment for their dependency.)

Scientists believe that the neurochemical dysfunction in addictions is best described as a chemical deficiency in one or more parts of the MFB. The chemicals speculated to be deficient are dopamine (best known to be increased in the ACC by cocaine), serotonin (5-hydroxytryptamine, 5-HT), endorphins, and gamma-aminobutyric acid (GABA). Thus, we can think of addictions as chemical deficiency diseases, much like Parkinsonism (caused by insufficient dopamine in a part of the brain) and diabetes, in which there is a lack of proper insulin release in the pancreas.

In a psychiatric sense, drug dependencies may be nothing more than sophisticated obsessive-compulsive disorders directed at particular favorite agents: alcohol, sex, food, gambling, overwork, cocaine, nicotine, etc. Some socially-sensitive scientists like this idea, since the negative public attitude toward drug addicts and alcoholics is so severe that funding for treatment, research, education, and prevention of these drug-induced diseases is miserably deficient. When people stop blaming the drug-afflicted for their disease by shifting the emphasis of blame from the drug to a brain-chemistry dysfunction leading to an inability to stop, perhaps public sympathy will produce a realistic movement to help those afflicted and suffering individuals with these diseases. But it will take time.

CONCLUSIONS

New findings in addiction science are telling us that drug dependence (addiction) is a disease over which the individual has no control. The disease process is best characterized as a brain chemistry-deficiency disorder, which will some day yield to much more cost-effective and specific therapies for addictions than those available today. Drug abuse (misuse) is a behavioral problem that responds to coercion, education, and decreased availability, whereas drug addictions require intensive multidimensional therapies that will soon include, and perhaps one day be replaced by, drug therapies discovered through new methods in neuropharmacology.

Notes

Chapter 2

1. Nauta, W. and Feirtag, M. (1986). *Fundamental neuroanatomy*, NY: Freeman, p. 309.

Chapter 3

1. Brick, J. (1987). *Drugs and the brain. An introduction to neuropharmacology.* New Brunswick, NJ: Rutgers University Center of Alcohol Studies.
2. Watson, P. (1989). Total body water and blood alcohol levels: Updating the fundamentals. In: K. Crow and R. Batt (Eds.), *Human metabolism of alcohol,* Boca Raton, FL: CRC Press, pp. 41-58.

Chapter 6

1. Johnson, L., O'Malley, P., and Bachman, J. (1996). Monitoring the future study 1975-1996. Rockville, MD: USDHHS, National Institute on Drug Abuse.
2. *Diagnostic and Statistical Manual of Mental Disorders*, Fourth Edition. (1994). Washington, DC: American Psychiatric Association.
3. Frezza, M., DiPadova, C., Pozzato, G., Terpin, M., Baraona, E., and Lieber, C. S. (1990). High blood alcohol levels in women: The role of decreased gastric alcohol dehydrogenase activity and first-pass metabolism, *New England Journal of Medicine,* 322(2), pp. 95-99.
4. Davenport, H. (1971). *Physiology of the digestive tract,* Chicago: Yearbook Medical Publishers, pp. 163-173.
5. Pohorecky, L., and Brick, J. (1990). The pharmacology of ethanol. In: *International encyclopedia of pharmacological therapeutics: Psychotropic drugs of abuse*, Elmsford, NY: Pergamon Press, pp. 189-254.
6. Widmark, E. (1981). *Principles and application of medicolegal alcohol determination,* CA: Biomedical Publications, pp. 47-82.
7. Center of Alcohol Studies, Rutgers University (1980). *Alco-calculator,* Alco-Research Documentation, Inc. New Brunswick, NJ: Author.
8. Many researchers, including the first author, have observed this in the laboratory. The strong central tendency of this rate of elimination is derived from data on variance. For example, Dubowski, K. (1985), Absorption, distribution

and elimination of alcohol: Highway safety aspects, *Journal of Studies on Alcohol*, 10, pp. 98-108, Table 2, reported a mean rate of alcohol elimination of 14.94 mg/dl/hr (.01494 percent/hr + .39 s.e.m.).

9. Palmer, R. (1994). Cimetidine and alcohol, *Drug Investigation*, 8(1), pp. 63-65.

10. Brick, J., Adler, J., Cocco, K., and Westrick, E. (1992). Alcohol intoxication: Pharmacokinetic prediction and behavioral analysis, *Current Topics in Pharmacology*, 1, pp. 57-67.

11. Ibid.

12. See Note 6 above.

13. Cocco, K., Adler, J., Westrick, E., Nathan, P., and Brick, J. (1986). Computerized program for the calculation of target blood alcohol levels in humans, *Proceedings and Abstracts of the Eastern Psychological Association*, 57, p. 29.

14. Brick, J. (1991, revised 1994). *Driving while intoxicated,* New Brunswick, NJ: Rutgers University Center of Alcohol Studies.

Chapter 7

1. Johnson, L., O'Malley, P., and Bachman, J. (1996). Monitoring the future study 1975-1996. Rockville, MD: USDHHS, National Institute on Drug Abuse.

2. Giros, B., Jaber, M., Jones, S., Wightman, R., and Caron, M. (1996). Hyperlocomotion and indifference to cocaine and amphetamine in mice lacking the dopamine transporter, *Nature,* 379, pp. 606-612.

3. Lakosko, J., Gallaway, M., and White, F. (Eds.) (1992). *Cocaine Pharmacology, Physiology and Clinical Strategies,* Boca Raton, FL: CRC Press, pp. 372-373.

4. Langenbucher, J., McCrady, B., Brick, J., and Esterly, R. (1993). Socioeconomic evaluations of addictions treatment, President's Commission on Model State Drug Laws, Washington, DC: The White House.

5. Hutchings, D. (1993). The puzzle of cocaine's effects following maternal use during pregnancy: Are there reconcilable differences? *Neurotoxiocology and Teratology*, 15, pp. 281-286.

6. See Note 2 above.

Chapter 8

1. Swonger, A. and Constantine, L. (1983). *Drugs and therapy,* Boston/Toronto: Little, Brown.

Chapter 9

1. Phillips, L. (1985). *Drug law enforcement training manual*, South Carolina Justice Academy.

2. Johnston, L., O'Malley, P., and Bachman, J. (1996). Monitoring the future study 1975-1996. Rockville, MD: USDHHS, National Institute on Drug Abuse.

3. Howlett, A., Egans, D., and Houston, D. (1992). The cannabinoid receptor. In: L. Murphy and A. Bartke (Eds.), *Marijuana/cannabinoids: Neurobiology and neurophysiology*, Boca Raton, FL: CRC Press, pp. 35-72.

4. Ibid.

5. Modified from Note 2.

6. Chait, L. and Pierri, J. (1992). Effects of smoked marijuana on human performance: A critical review. In: L. Murphy and A. Bartke (Eds.), *Marijuana/cannabinoids: Neurobiology and neurophysiology*, Boca Raton, FL: CRC Press, pp. 387-423.

7. Yesavage, J., Leirer, V., and Denari, M. (1985). Carry-over effects of marijuana intoxication on aircraft pilot performance: A preliminary report, *American Journal of Psychiatry*, 142, p. 1325.

8. Ray, O. S. and Ksir, C. (1987). *Drugs, society and human behavior*, fourth edition, St. Louis: Times Mirror/Mosby College Publishing, pp. 300-321.

Chapter 10

1. Darwin, C. (1872). *The expression of emotions in man and animals.* London: John Murry.

Chapter 11

1. Schildkraut, J. (1965). The catecholamine hypothesis of affective disorders: A review of supporting evidence. *American Journal of Psychiatry*, 122, pp. 509-522.

Chapter 12

1. Pinel, J. (1989). *Biopsychology.* Needham Heights, MA: Allyn & Bacon.

2. Chiodo, L. A. and Bunney, B. S. (1987). Population response of midbrain dopaminergic neurons to neuroleptics: Further studies on time course and non-dopaminergic neuronal influences, *Journal of Neuroscience*, 7, pp. 629-633.

Chapter 13

1. *Diagnostic and Statistical Manual of Mental Disorders*, Fourth Edition. (1994). Washington, DC: American Psychiatric Association.

2. Robinson, T. E. and Berridge, K. C. (1993). The neural basis of drug craving: An incentive sensitization theory of addiction. *Brain Research Review*, 18, pp. 246-291.

Selected Bibliography

Chapter 2

Clark, J. (Ed.) (1984). *The human body: The brain: Mystery of matter and mind,* New York: Torstar Books.

Clark, J. (Ed.) (1984). *The human body: The nervous system,* New York: Torstar Books.

Glickman, S. E. and Schiff, B. B. (1967). A biological theory of reinforcement, *Psychological Reviews,* 74: 81-109.

Gregory, R. (Ed.) (1987). *The Oxford companion to the mind,* New York: Oxford University Press.

Koob, G. F. (1992). Neural mechanisms of drug reinforcement. In: P. Kalivas and H. Samson (Eds.), *The neurobiology of drug and alcohol addiction,* Vol. 654, Annals of the American Academy of Sciences, pp. 171-191.

Nauta, W. and Feirtag, M. (1986). *Fundamental neuroanatomy,* New York: Freeman, p. 309.

Olds, J. and Milner, P. (1954). Positive reinforcement produced by electrical stimulation of the septal area and other regions of the rat brain, *Journal of Comparative and Physiological Psychology,* 47: pp. 419-427.

Wise, R. (1990). The role of reward pathways in the development of drug dependence. In: D. Balfour (Ed.), *Psychotropic drugs of abuse,* Elmsford, NY: Pergamon Press.

Chapter 3

Benet, L., Mitchell, J. and Sheiner, L. (1990). Pharmacokinetics: The dynamics of drug absorption, distribution and elimination. In: L. Goodman and A. Gilman (Eds.), *The pharmacological basis of therapeutics,* New York: McGraw-Hill, pp. 3-32.

Brick, J. (1987). *Drugs and the brain,* New Brunswick, NJ: Rutgers University Center of Alcohol Studies.

Watson, P. Total body water and blood alcohol levels: Updating the fundamentals. In: K. Crow and R. Batt (Eds.), *Human metabolism of alcohol,* Vol. 1, Boca Raton, FL: CRC Press, pp. 41-58.

Chapter 4

Carpenter, M. (1976). *Human neuroanatomy,* Baltimore: Williams and Wilkins.

Pinel, J. (1990). *Biopsychology,* Needham Heights, MA: Allyn and Bacon.

Chapter 5

Brick, J. (1987). *Drugs and the brain*, New Brunswick, NJ: Rutgers University Center of Alcohol Studies.

Diem, K. and Lentner, C. (1971). Scientific tables. Basle, Switzerland: Ciba-Geisn, Ltd., p. 516.

Wilcox, R. E. and Gonzales, R. A. (1995). Introduction to neurotransmitters, receptors, signal transduction and second messengers. In: A. F. Schatzberg and C. B. Nemeroff (Eds.), *Textbook of Psychopharmacology*, Washington, DC: American Psychiatric Press, Inc., pp. 3-30.

Chapter 6

Brick, J. (1991, revised 1994). *Driving while intoxicated*, New Brunswick, NJ: Rutgers University Center of Alcohol Studies.

Brick, J. (1995). *Fetal alcohol and drug effects*, New Brunswick, NJ: Rutgers University Center of Alcohol Studies.

Brick, J., Adler, J., Cocco, K., and Westrick, E. (1992). Alcohol intoxication: Pharmacokinetic prediction and behavioral analysis, *Current Topics in Pharmacology* 1, pp. 57-67.

Center of Alcohol Studies. (1980). *Alco-calculator*, Alco-Research Documentation, Inc. New Brunswick, NJ: Rutgers University Center of Alcohol Studies.

Cocco, K., Adler, J. Westrick, E., Nathan, P., and Brick, J. (1986). Computerized program for the calculation of target blood alcohol levels in humans, *Proceedings and Abstracts of the Annual Meeting of the Eastern Psychological Association,* 57, p. 29.

Davenport, H. (1971). *Physiology of the digestive tract,* Chicago: Yearbook Medical Publishers, pp. 163-173.

Diagnostic and statistical manual of mental disorders, Fourth Edition. (1994). Washington, DC: American Psychiatric Association.

Dubowski, K. M. (1985). Absorption, distribution and elimination of alcohol: Highway safety aspects. *Journal on Studies of Alcohol Supplement,* 10, pp. 98-108.

Frezza, M., DiPadova, C., Pozzato, G., Terpin, M., Baraona, E., and Lieber, C. S. (1990). High blood alcohol levels in women: The role of decreased gastric alcohol dehydrogenase activity and first-pass metabolism, *New England Journal of Medicine,* 322(2), pp. 95-99.

Haggard, H. W., Greenberg, L. A., and Cohen, L. H. (1938). Quantitative differences in the effects of alcoholic beverages, *New England Journal of Medicine* 219, pp. 446-470.

Harger, R. N. and Forney, R. B. (1963). Aliphatic alcohols. In: A. Stolman (Ed.), *Progress in chemical toxicology*, New York: Academic Press, p. 79.

Hendrix, T. (1974). The motility of the alimentary canal. In: V. B. Mountcastle (Ed.), *Medical physiology,* Vol. 2, St. Louis, MO: C. V. Mosby, pp. 1208-1236.

Johnson, L., O'Malley, P., and Bachman, J. (1996). Monitoring the future study 1975-1996. Rockville, MD: USDHHS, National Institute on Drug Abuse.

Kalant, H. (1971). Absorption, diffusion, distribution an elimination of ethanol: Effects on biological membranes. In: B. Kissin and H. Begleiter (Eds.), *The biology of alcoholism*, Vol. 1, *Biochemistry*, New York: Plenum Press, pp. 1-46.

Langenbucher, J., McCrady, B., Brick, J., and Esterly, R. (1993). *Socioeconomic evaluations of addictions treatment*, Washington, DC: The White House, President's Commission on Model State Drug Laws.

Niaura, R. S., Nathan, P. E., Frankenstein, W., Shapiro, A. P., and Brick, J. (1987). Gender differences in acute psychomotor, cognitive, and pharmacokinetic response to alcohol, *Addictive Behaviors*, 12, pp. 345-356.

Palmer, R. (1994). Cimetidine and alcohol, *Drug Investigation*, 8(1), pp. 63-65.

Pohorecky, L. and Brick, J. (1990). The pharmacology of ethanol. In: D. Balfour (Ed.), *International encyclopedia of pharmacological therapeutics: Psychotropic drugs of abuse*, Elmsford, NY: Pergamon Press, pp. 189-254.

Von Wartburg, J. (1989). Pharmacokinetics of alcohol. In: K. P. Crow and R. P. Batt (Eds.), *Human metabolism of alcohol*, Boca Raton, FL: CRC Press, pp. 9-22.

Watson, P. E. (1989). Total body water and blood alcohol levels: Updating the fundamentals. In: K. Crow and R. Batt (Eds.), *Human metabolism of alcohol*, Boca Raton, FL: CRC Press, pp. 41-58.

Widmark, E. (1981). *Principles and application of medicolegal alcohol determination*, CA: Biomedical Publications, pp. 47-82.

Wilkinson, P. K. (1980). Pharmacokinetics of ethanol: A review, *Alcoholism: Clinical and Experimental Research*, 4, pp. 6-21.

Wilson, G. T., Brick, J., Adler, J., Cocco, K., and Breslin, C. (1989). Alcohol and anxiety reduction in female social drinkers, *Journal of Studies on Alcohol* 50(3), pp. 226-335.

Chapter 7

Barnes, D. (1988). The biological tangle of drug addiction, *Science,* 241, pp. 415-417.

Barnes, D. (1988). Drugs: Running the numbers, *Science,* 240, pp. 1729-1731.

Brick, J. (1988). *Drugs and the brain: An introduction to neuropharmacology.* New Brunswick, NJ: Rutgers University Center of Alcohol Studies Publication Division.

Brown, R. (1989). Pharmacology of cocaine abuse. In: K. K. Redda, C. A. Walker, and G. Barnett (Eds.), *Cocaine, marijuana, designer drugs: Chemistry and pharmacology*, Boca Raton, FL: CRC Press, pp. 39-52.

Byck, R. (1987). The effects of cocaine on complex performance in humans, *Alcohol, Drugs and Driving* 3(1): pp. 9-12.

Clouet, D., Asghar, K., and Brown, R. (1988). *Mechanisms of cocaine abuse and toxicity*, Rockville, MD: National Institute on Drug Abuse, NIDA Research Monograph 88.

Giros, B., Jaber, M., Jones, S., Wightman, R., and Caron, M. (1996). Hyperlocomotion and indifference to cocaine and amphetamine in mice lacking the dopamine transporter, *Nature*, 379, pp. 606-612.

Hutchings, D. (1993). The puzzle of cocaine's effects following maternal use during pregnancy: Are there reconcilable differences? *Neurotoxicology and Teratology*, (15), pp. 281-286.

Johnson, L., O'Malley, P., and Bachman, J. (1996). Monitoring the future study 1975-1996. Rockville, MD: USDHHS, National Institute on Drug Abuse.

Lakosko, J., Gallaway, M., and White, F. (Eds.) (1992). *Cocaine pharmacology, physiology and clinical strategies*, Boca Raton, FL: CRC Press, pp. 372-373.

Langenbucher, J., McCrady, B., Brick, J., and Esterly, R. (1993). Socioeconomic evaluations of addictions treatment, President's Commission on Model State Drug Laws, Washington, DC: The White House.

Siegel, R. K. (1987). Cocaine use and driving behavior, *Alcohol, Drugs and Driving*, 3(1), pp. 1-7.

Widmark, E. (1981). *Principles and application of medicolegal alcohol determination*, CA: Biomedical Publications, pp. 47-82.

Chapter 8

Bloom, F. E. (1983). The endorphins. A growing family of pharmacologically pertinent peptides, *Annual Review of Pharmacology and Toxicology*, pp. 151-170.

Jaffe, J. and Martin, W. (1975). Narcotic analgesics and antagonists. In: L. Goodman and A. Gilman (Eds.), *Pharmacological basis of therapeutics*, New York: Macmillan, pp. 245-283.

Swonger, A. and Constantine, L. (1983). *Drugs and therapy*, Boston: Little, Brown.

Chapter 9

Agurel, S. L. and Hollister, L. E. (1986). Pharmacokinetics and metabolism of delta-9-tetrahydrocannabinol: Relations to effects in man, *Alcohol, Drugs and Driving*, 2: pp. 61-77.

Brick, J. (1990). *Marijuana*, New Brunswick, NJ: Rutgers University Center of Alcohol Studies.

Canavan, D. I. (1987). Screening: Urine drug tests. *Maryland Medical Journal*, 36, pp. 229-233.

Chait, L. and Pierri, J. (1992). Effect of smoked marijuana on human performance: A critical review. In: L. Murphy and A. Bartke (Eds.), *Marijuana/cannabinoids: Neurobiology and neurophysiology*, Boca Raton, FL: CRC Press, pp. 387-425.

Chiang, C. N. and Rapaka, R. S. (1987). Pharmacokinetics and disposition of cannabinoids. In: R. S. Rapaka and A. Makriyannis (Eds.), *Structure-activity relationships of the cannabinoids*, Rockville, MD: National Institute on Drug Abuse, U.S. Department of Health and Human Services, Research Monograph 79.

Department of Health and Human Services (1987). *Drug abuse and drug abuse research: Marijuana and cannabinoids. The second triennial report to con-*

gress *from the secretary, Department of Health and Human Services*, ADAMHA, NIAAA. Rockville, MD: Author, pp. 77-91.

Ellis, G. M., Mann, M. A., Judson, B. A., Schramm, N. T., and Taschian, A. (1985). Excretion patterns of cannabinoid metabolites after last use in a group of chronic users, *Clinical Pharmacology of Therapeutics*, 38, pp. 572-578.

Erickson, C. (1992). A comment on marijuana and a recent paper, *Science Matters*, 2(6), pp. 21, 24.

Fehr O'Brien, K. and Kalant, H. (1983). Cannabis and health hazards. *Proceeding of an Addiction Research Foundation/World Health Organization scientific meeting on adverse health and behavioral consequences of cannabis use*, Toronto: Addiction Research Foundation.

Howlett, A., Egans, D., and Houston, D. (1992). The cannabinoid receptor. In: L. Murphy and A. Bartke (Eds.), *Marijuana/cannabinoids: Neurobiology and neurophysiology*, Boca Raton, FL: CRC Press, pp. 35-72.

Johnston, L. D., O'Malley, P. M., and Bachman, J. G. (1988). *Illicit drug use, smoking, and drinking by America's high school students, college students and young adults: 1975-1987*. National Institute on Drug Abuse, U.S. Department of Health and Human Services Publication No. (ADM) 89-1602, Washington, DC: U.S. Government Printing Office.

Johnston, L., O'Malley, P., and Bachman, J. (1996). *Monitoring the future study 1975-1996*, Rockville, MD: National Institute on Drug Abuse, U.S. Department of Health and Human Services.

New York Times Magazine (February 19, 1995). Marijuana in the 1990s. Section 6.

Phillips, L. (1985). Drug law enforcement training manual. South Carolina Criminal Justice Academy.

Ray, O. S. and Ksir, C. (1987). *Drugs, society and human behavior*, fourth edition, St. Louis: Times Mirror/Mosby College Publishing, pp. 300-321.

Schuckit, M. A. (1989). Cannabinols. In: M. A. Schuckit (Ed.), *Drug and alcohol abuse: A clinical guide to diagnosis and treatment*, New York: Plenum Medical Book Co., pp. 143-157.

Smiley, A. (1986). Marijuana: On-road and driving simulator studies, *Alcohol, Drugs and Driving*, 2(3-4), pp. 121-134.

Wu, T. C., Tashkin, O. P., Djahed, B., and Rose, J. E. (1988). Pulmonary hazards of smoking marijuana as compared with tobacco, *New England Journal of Medicine*, 318, pp. 347-351.

Yesavage, J., Leirer, V., Denari, M., and Hollister, L. (1985). Carry-over effects of marijuana intoxication on aircraft pilot performance: A preliminary report, *American Journal of Psychiatry*, 142, pp. 1325-1329.

Chapter 10

Ballenger, J. (1995). Benzodiazepines. In: A. Schatzberg and C. Nemeroff (Eds.), *Textbook of psychopharmacology*, Washington, DC: American Psychiatric Press, pp. 215-230.

Brick, J. and Pohorecky, L. A. (Eds.) (1983). *Stress and alcohol use*, New York: Elsevier Biomedical, pp. 389-402.

Darwin, C. (1872). *The expression of emotions in man and animals.* London: John Murry.

Chapter 11

Charney, D. S., Miller, H. L., Licinio, J., and Salomon, K. (1995). Treatment of depression. In: A. Schatzberg and C. Nemeroff (Eds.), *Textbook of psychopharmacology*, Washington, DC: American Psychiatric Press, pp. 575-602.
Feldman, R. S. and Quenzer, L. F. (1984). *Fundamentals of neuropsychopharmacology*, Sunderland, MA: Sinauer Associates, pp. 369-398.
Potter, W., Manji, H., and Rudorfer, M. (1995). Tricyclics and tetracyclics. In: A. Schatzberg and C. Nemeroff (Eds.), *Textbook of psychopharmacology*, Washington, DC: American Psychiatric Press, pp. 141-160.
Schildkraut (1965). The catecholamine hypothesis of affective disorders: A review of supporting evidence. *American Journal of Psychiatry*, 122, pp. 509-522.
Stahl, S. M. and Palazidon, L. (1986). The pharmacology of depression, *Trends in Pharmacological Sciences,* 7, pp. 349-354.

Chapter 12

Bach-y-Rita, P. (1994). Psychopharmacologic drugs: Mechanisms of action, *Science*, 264, pp. 642-643.
Baldessarino, R. (1990). Drugs and the treatment of psychiatric disorders. In: L. Goodman and A. Gilman (Eds.), *The pharmacological basis of therapeutics*, eighth edition, New York: McGraw-Hill, pp. 383-435.
Buckley, P. and Meltzer, H. (1995). Treatment of schizophrenia. In: A. Schatzberg and C. Nemeroff (Eds.), *Textbook of psychopharmacology*, Washington, DC: American Psychiatric Press, pp. 615-640.
Chiodo, L. A. and Bunney, B. S. (1987). Population response of midbrain dopaminergic neurons to neuroleptics: Further studies on time course and nondopaminergic neuronal influences, *Journal of Neuroscience,* 7, pp. 629-633.
Farde, L., Nordstrom, A. L., Wiesel, F. A., Pauli, S., Halldin, C., and Sedvall, G. (1992). Positron emission tomographic analysis of central D1 and D2 dopamine receptor occupancy in patients treated with classical neuroleptics and clozapine, *Archives of General Psychiatry*, 49, pp. 538-544.
Green, A. I. and Salzman, C. (1990). Clozapine: Benefits and risks, *Hospital and Community Psychiatry,* 41, pp. 379-380.
Hollandsworth, J. (1990). *The physiology of psychological disorders,* New York: Plenum Press.
Julien, R. (1992). *A primer of drug action*, New York: Freeman Press, pp. 215-238.
Marder, S. R., Wirshing, W., and Van Putten, T. (1991). Drug treatment of schizophrenia: Overview of recent research, *Schizophrenia Research,* 4, pp. 81-90.
Pinel, J. (1989). *Biopsychology,* Needham Heights, MA: Allyn & Bacon.

Chapter 13

Diagnostic and statistical manual of mental disorders, Fourth edition. (1994). Washington, DC: American Psychiatric Association.

Erickson, C. K. (1992). A pharmacologist's opinion. Alcoholism: The disease debate needs to stop, *Alcohol and Alcoholism,* 4, pp. 325-328.

Grant, B. F. and Pickering, R. P. (1996). Comorbidity between DSM-IV alcohol and drug use disorders, *Alcohol Health Research World,* 20, pp. 67-72.

Koob, G. F. (1992). Drugs of abuse: Anatomy, pharmacology and function of reward pathways, *Trends in Pharmacological Science,* 13, pp. 177-193.

Lewis, D. C. (1991). Comparison of alcoholism and other medical diseases: An internist's view, *Psychiatry Annals,* 21, pp. 256-265.

Robinson, T. E. and Berridge, K. C. (1993). The neural basis of drug craving: An incentive sensitization theory of addiction. *Brain Research Review,* 18, pp. 246-291.

Index

Order Your Own Copy of
This Important Book for Your Personal Library!

DRUGS, THE BRAIN, AND BEHAVIOR
The Pharmacology of Abuse and Dependence

_____ in hardbound at $49.95 (ISBN: 0-7890-0274-4)

COST OF BOOKS _____

OUTSIDE USA/CANADA/
MEXICO: ADD 20% _____

POSTAGE & HANDLING _____
(US: $3.00 for first book & $1.25
for each additional book)
Outside US: $4.75 for first book
& $1.75 for each additional book)

SUBTOTAL _____

IN CANADA: ADD 7% GST _____

STATE TAX _____
(NY, OH & MN residents, please
add appropriate local sales tax)

FINAL TOTAL _____
(If paying in Canadian funds,
convert using the current
exchange rate. UNESCO
coupons welcome.)

☐ **BILL ME LATER:** ($5 service charge will be added)
(Bill-me option is good on US/Canada/Mexico orders only;
not good to jobbers, wholesalers, or subscription agencies.)

☐ Check here if billing address is different from
shipping address and attach purchase order and
billing address information.

Signature _____

☐ **PAYMENT ENCLOSED: $** _____

☐ **PLEASE CHARGE TO MY CREDIT CARD.**

☐ Visa   ☐ MasterCard   ☐ AmEx   ☐ Discover
☐ Diners Club
Account # _____

Exp. Date _____

Signature _____

Prices in US dollars and subject to change without notice.

NAME _____

INSTITUTION _____

ADDRESS _____

CITY _____

STATE/ZIP _____

COUNTRY _____ COUNTY (NY residents only) _____

TEL _____ FAX _____

E-MAIL_____
May we use your e-mail address for confirmations and other types of information? ☐ Yes   ☐ No

Order From Your Local Bookstore or Directly From
The Haworth Press, Inc.
10 Alice Street, Binghamton, New York 13904-1580 • USA
TELEPHONE: 1-800-HAWORTH (1-800-429-6784) / Outside US/Canada: (607) 722-5857
FAX: 1-800-895-0582 / Outside US/Canada: (607) 772-6362
E-mail: getinfo@haworth.com
PLEASE PHOTOCOPY THIS FORM FOR YOUR PERSONAL USE.

BOF96

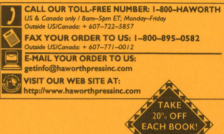
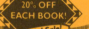